Advances in Minimally Invasive Surgery

Editor

ANTHONY PERERA

FOOT AND ANKLE CLINICS

www.foot.theclinics.com

Consulting Editor
MARK S. MYERSON

September 2020 • Volume 25 • Number 3

ELSEVIER

1600 John F. Kennedy Boulevard • Suite 1800 • Philadelphia, Pennsylvania, 19103-2899

http://www.theclinics.com

FOOT AND ANKLE CLINICS Volume 25, Number 3
September 2020 ISSN 1083-7515, ISBN-978-0-323-75909-0

Editor: Lauren Boyle
Developmental Editor: Nicole Congleton

Foot and Ankle Clinics (ISSN 1083-7515) is published quarterly by Elsevier, Inc., 360 Park Avenue South, New York, NY 10010-1710. Months of issue are March, June, September, and December. Periodicals postage paid at New York, NY, and additional mailing offices. Subscription price per year is $340.00 (US individuals), $582.00 (US institutions), $100.00 (US students), $371.00 (Canadian individuals), $669.00 (Canadian institutions), $100.00 (Canadian students), $470.00 (international individuals), $669.00 (international institutions), and $215.00 (international students). To receive student/resident rate, orders must be accompanied by name of affiliated institution, date of term, and the *signature* of program/residency coordinator on institution letterhead. Orders will be billed at individual rate until proof of status is received. Foreign air speed delivery is included in all *Clinics* subscription prices. All prices are subject to change without notice. **POSTMASTER:** Send address changes to *Foot and Ankle Clinics*, Elsevier Health Sciences Division, Subscription Customer Service, 3251 Riverport Lane, Maryland Heights, MO 63043. **Customer Service: 1-800-654-2452 (US and Canada). From outside of the United States and Canada, call 314-447-8871. Fax: 314-447-8029. E-mail: JournalsCustomerService-usa@ elsevier.com (for print support); JournalsOnlineSupport-usa@elsevier.com (for online support).**

Reprints. For copies of 100 or more, of articles in this publication, please contact the Commercial Reprints Department, Elsevier Inc., 360 Park Avenue South, New York, NY 10010-1710. Tel.: 212-633-3874; Fax: 212-633-3820; E-mail: reprints@elsevier.com.

Contributors

CONSULTING EDITOR

MARK S. MYERSON, MD
Executive Director and Founder, Steps2Walk, Baltimore, Maryland, USA

EDITOR

ANTHONY PERERA, MBChB, MRCS, MFSEM (RCP & SI), FRCS (Orth)
University Hospital of Wales Llandough, University Hospital of Wales Cardiff, Spire Cardiff Hospital, Cardiff, Wales, United Kingdom

AUTHORS

HARVINDER BEDI, MBBS, MPH, FRACS
Department of Orthopaedic Surgery, Box Hill Hospital, Melbourne, Victoria, Australia

ALESSIO BERNASCONI, MD, PhD, FEBOT
Department of Public Health, Trauma and Orthopaedics, University of Naples Federico II, Naples, Italy; Foot and Ankle Unit, Royal National Orthopaedic Hospital, Stanmore, United Kingdom

CARLO BIZ, MD
Associate Professor, Department of Surgery, Oncology and Gastroenterology DiSCOG, Orthopedic and Traumatologic Clinic, University of Padova, Padova, Italy; GRECMIP-MIFAS (Groupe de Recherche et d'Etude en Chirurgie Mini-Invasive du Pied-Minimally Invasive Foot and Ankle Society), Merignac, France

GUILLAUME CORDIER, MD
Clinique du Sport Bordeaux-Mérignac, France; GRECMIP-MIFAS (Group of Research and Study in Minimally Invasive Surgery of the Foot–Minimally Invasive Foot and Ankle Society), Merignac, France

MIKI DALMAU-PASTOR, PhD
Human Anatomy Unit, Department of Pathology and Experimental Therapeutics, School of Medicine and Health Sciences, University of Barcelona, Barcelona, Spain; GRECMIP - MIFAS (Groupe de Recherche et d'Etude en Chirurgie Mini-Invasive du Pied - Minimally Invasive Foot and Ankle Society), Merignac, France

JORGE JAVIER DEL VECCHIO, MD, MBA
GRECMIP - MIFAS (Groupe de Recherche et d'Etude en Chirurgie Mini-Invasive du Pied - Minimally Invasive Foot and Ankle Society), Merignac, France; Head, Foot and Ankle Section, Orthopaedics Department, Fundación Favaloro -Hospital Universitario, Ciudad Autónoma de Buenos Aires (CABA), Argentina; Department of Kinesiology and Physiatry, Universidad Favaloro, CABA, Argentina

STÉPHANE GUILLO, MD
Orthopaedic Surgeon, Orthopaedic Department, Mérignac Sport Clinic, Mérignac, France

BEN HICKEY, BM, MRCS, MSc, FRCS (Tr & Orth), MD
Department of Orthopaedic Surgery, Wrexham Maelor Hospital, Wrexham, Wales

GEORG HOCHHEUSER, MD
Chirurgisch Orthopädisches Centrum am diako, Augsburg, Germany; GRECMIP soon
MIFAS: Minimally Invasive Foot and Ankle Society, Merignac, France; GFFC: German
Society of Foot and Ankle Surgery, Raisting, Germany

LUCKSHMANA JEYASEELAN, MBBS, BSc, FRCS (Tr&Orth)
Locum Consultant Orthopaedic Foot and Ankle Surgeon, The Foot and Ankle Unit,
Department of Trauma and Orthopaedics, Barts Health NHS Trust, The Royal London
Hospital, London, United Kindom

DAVID B. KAY, MD
Professor Orthopedic Surgery, Northeast Ohio Medical University, Akron, Ohio, USA

ANDREW KING, MBChB, MRCS
ST6 Specialty Registrar, Trauma and Orthopaedics Department, Royal Cornwall
Hospitals NHS Trust, Royal Cornwall Hospital, Truro, United Kingdom

ANNA-KATHRIN LEUCHT, MD
Footbridge Centre for Integrated Orthopaedic Care, Providence Health Care, Vancouver,
British Columbia, Canada; Department of Orthopaedics and Traumatology, Cantonal
Hospital of Winterthur, Switzerland

FRANCESC MALAGELADA, MD, FEBOT, PhD
Consultant Orthopaedic Foot and Ankle Surgeon, The Foot and Ankle Unit, Department of
Trauma and Orthopaedics, Barts Health NHS Trust, The Royal London Hospital, London,
United Kingdom

FREDERICK MICHELS, MD
Orthopaedic Department, AZ Groeninge, Kortrijk, Belgium; Ankle Instability Group,
GRECMIP - MIFAS (Groupe de Recherche et d'Etude en Chirurgie Mini-Invasive du Pied -
Minimally Invasive Foot and Ankle Society), Merignac, France

GUSTAVO ARAUJO NUNES, MD
GRECMIP-MIFAS (Group of Research and Study in Minimally Invasive Surgery of the
Foot–Minimally Invasive Foot and Ankle Society), Merignac, France; Hospital Ortopédico,
Belo Horizonte, Minas Gerais, Brazil

STEPHEN PARSONS, MA, BS, FRCS, FRCS (Ed)
Consultant Foot and Ankle Surgeon, Trauma and Orthopaedics Department, Royal
Cornwall Hospitals NHS Trust, Royal Cornwall Hospital, Truro, United Kingdom

ANTHONY PERERA, MBChB, MRCS, MFSEM (RCP & SI), FRCS (Orth)
University Hospital of Wales Llandough, University Hospital of Wales Cardiff, Spire Cardiff
Hospital, Cardiff, Wales, United Kingdom

ROBBIE RAY, MB ChB, ChM(T&O), FRCSed(T&O), FEBOT
Princess Royal University Hospital, King's College Hospital NHS Foundation Trust,
Orpington, London, United Kingdom

DAVID REDFERN, MBBS, FRCS
Montefiore Hospital, Hove, East Sussex, England; London Foot and Ankle Centre,
Hospital of St John and St Elizabeth, London, England

PIETRO RUGGIERI, MD, PhD
Full Professor, Department of Surgery, Oncology and Gastroenterology DiSCOG,
Orthopedic and Traumatologic Clinic, University of Padova, Padova, Italy

ANDREA VELJKOVIC, MD, MPH(Harvard), BComm, FAOA, FRCSC
Footbridge Centre for Integrated Orthopaedic Care, Providence Health Care, University of
British Columbia, Vancouver, British Columbia, Canada

JOEL VERNOIS, MD
Sussex Orthopaedic NHS Treatment Centre, Haywards Heath, West Sussex, England;
ICP, Clinique Blomet, Paris, France

ALASTAIR YOUNGER, MB ChB, MSc, ChM, FRCSC
Footbridge Centre for Integrated Orthopaedic Care, Providence Health Care, Vancouver,
British Columbia, Canada

Editorial Advisory Board

Contents

tendons will re-align once the bone deformity is corrected. The periosteum is maintained to provide a biologic scaffold for new bone formation and must be minimally disrupted during the intervention.

Complications of Minimally Invasive Surgery for Hallux Valgus and How to Deal with Them

Georg Hochheuser

This article discusses the possible complications in minimally invasive surgery (MIS) for hallux valgus. The rate of complications and the outcomes are at least comparable with open techniques. A percutaneous technique provides the best conditions for undisturbed healing. Some possible complications exist in MIS that do not exist in open surgery, such as lesion of soft tissue structures that are not under direct visible control or skin burns. These complications usually result from technical mistakes in performing the operation. It is therefore crucial to get proper education from cadaver training and visiting experienced colleagues, as is done in open surgery.

Lapidus, a Percutaneous Approach

Joel Vernois, David Redfern and GRECMIP soon MIFAS

Described in the early 1900s by Albrecht and Lapidus, the Lapidus procedure became an important tool in the armamentarium. With the increase of percutaneous techniques, the development of a percutaneous Lapidus seemed obvious.

The Windswept Foot: Dealing with Metatarsus Adductus and Toe Valgus

Anna-Kathrin Leucht, Alastair Younger, Andrea Veljkovic, and Anthony Perera

The windswept foot remains a reconstructive challenge. The hallux valgus associated with the medially displaced lesser metatarsal heads is hard to correct. Either the lesser metatarsal heads need to be displaced laterally or the deformity accepted. With the deformity, all the toes tend to be aligned into valgus with the position of the flexor and extensor tendons. Several treatment alternatives exist and may require a combination of open and percutaneous surgery. The authors think that, in severe metatarsus adductus, proximal correction of the first, second, and third metatarsals is required.

Bunionette: Is There a Minimally Invasive Solution?

Frederick Michels and Stéphane Guillo

A bunionette deformity is a painful prominence on the lateral aspect of the fifth metatarsal head. Surgical treatment can be considered if conservative treatment has failed to relieve the symptoms. The percutaneous approach consists of 2 steps: a condylectomy and an osteotomy of the fifth metatarsal. The learning curve is small and the final results are similar to the open techniques. The main advantages are the hardware-free technique and the minimally invasive approach. This percutaneous approach avoids complications related to hardware and soft tissue healing. Because of this low complication rate, the percutaneous technique may become the new gold standard.

Video content accompanies this article at http://www.foot.theclinics. com.

Minimally invasive distal metatarsal diaphyseal osteotomy (DMDO) is an effective procedure for the treatment of complicated chronic diabetic foot ulcers under the heads of all lateral metatarsal bones (including the fifth). Resistant toe ulcers and recurrent pressure ulcers can be treated effectively by DMDO. For diabetic patients, the main advantages of this method are minimal surgical scars and tissue damage, immediately postoperative weight bearing, absence of osteosynthesis and consequent potential infection of metal fixation, reduction of the previous high plantar pressures by the restoration of a harmonic balanced forefoot arch, and rapid ulcer healing.

Minimally invasive procedures to treat lesser toes deformities are among the main surgeries of percutaneous techniques and considered mature techniques due to technical versatility and high correction potential, with low rates of complications. Although they seem technically simple procedures, there are important technical details for each of them to obtain a reliable correction. To achieve success in lesser toes percutaneous treatment, it is imperative to follow minimally invasive basic principles, especially postoperative care with specific bandages for unfixed osteotomies. Practical training is mandatory before starting the experience; the foot surgeon must learn theoretic and practical aspects to master this surgery.

Adult acquired flatfoot deformity (AAFD) as a consequence of posterior tibial tendon dysfunction is commonly divided in flexible (stages I and II) and fixed (stages III and IV) deformities. The aim of this article is to summarize the evidence available for minimally invasive surgical techniques that can be used in the treatment of flexible AAFD, including tibialis posterior tendoscopy, subtalar arthroereisis, minimally invasive calcaneal osteotomy, and medial proximal gastrocnemius recession. A treatment algorithm and technical tips have also been provided.

Endoscopic resection of tarsal coalitions is technically feasible for both talocalcaneal and calcaneonavicular coalitions. Careful consideration of each individual patient is necessary before proceeding with endoscopic resection. Endoscopic resection of these coalitions may offer benefits in terms of faster recovery and less wound problems, but this has not been proven. Several case reports and case series appear in the literature and are reviewed here along with the different techniques reported. Better-quality evidence is required to assess the clinically relevant benefits and the recurrence rate for endoscopic resection in comparison with open resection.

FOOT AND ANKLE CLINICS

RELATED SERIES

Clinics in Sports Medicine
Orthopedic Clinics
Physical Medicine and Rehabilitation Clinics

THE CLINICS ARE NOW AVAILABLE ONLINE!
Access your subscription at:
www.theclinics.com

Preface

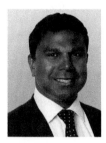

Anthony Perera, MBChB, MRCS,
MFSEM (RCP & SI), FRCS (Orth)
Editor

The first issue of *Foot and Ankle Clinics* devoted to minimally invasive techniques was published in 2016, and the first American Orthopaedic Foot & Ankle Society presentation on minimally invasive surgery (MIS) surgery was presented back in 2013 when I presented my 2 years of comparative results. We have come a long way since then. In that time percutaneous surgery has been introduced to North America, and there are now a number of highly skilled experts doing tremendous work there. This has gone on to become a popular procedure in the United States and Canada now thanks to GRECMIP, who have been instrumental in spreading this around the world through their training courses.

The debate has now moved on from the concept of MIS itself, and therefore, in this issue, we have focused on more of the technical aspects of practice. In the last preface, I called for the development of new procedures and implants to maximize the advantages of percutaneous surgery so that we could continue to move away from simply trying to do existing procedures through a smaller incision. This development has occurred on pace. We present some of these techniques here, and there are many more to come.

This issue reflects the global nature of interest in percutaneous, endoscopic, and arthroscopic foot surgery with authors from all around the world. I would like to thank them for their time and for sharing their knowledge so that we can all benefit from the rapid developments that have occurred. Finally, I must send a huge thanks to the staff

Foot Ankle Clin N Am 25 (2020) xiii–xiv
https://doi.org/10.1016/j.fcl.2020.07.001
1083-7515/20/© 2020 Published by Elsevier Inc.

foot.theclinics.com

at Elsevier, who has worked so hard to deliver this project, and Dr Mark Myerson, my friend and mentor, for giving me this opportunity.

Anthony Perera, MBChB, MRCS, MFSEM (RCP & SI), FRCS (Orth)
University Hospital of Wales Llandough
University Hospital of Wales Cardiff
Spire Cardiff Hospital
Croescadaran Road
Cardiff, Wales CF23 8XL, UK

E-mail address:
footandanklesurgery@gmail.com

Minimally Invasive Hallux Valgus Surgery—A Systematic Review and Assessment of State of the Art

Luckshmana Jeyaseelan, MBBS, BSc, FRCS (Tr&Orth),
Francesc Malagelada, MD, FEBOT, PhD*

KEYWORDS

- Hallux valgus • Minimally invasive • Percutaneous • MIS • MICA

KEY POINTS

- Minimally invasive surgery in the treatment of hallux valgus is a safe and effective technique.
- Radiological and clinical outcomes seem to be comparative to open procedures.
- There is currently insufficient evidence to recommend minimally invasive surgery over open procedures for the correction of hallux valgus.
- There is currently insufficient evidence to recommend one minimally invasive technique over another.
- There is a need for prospective, randomized studies focusing on comparing minimally invasive techniques to both open techniques and to other minimally invasive techniques.

INTRODUCTION

Hallux valgus is a common deformity, with epidemiologic studies suggesting a prevalence of between 23% and 35.7%.[1–3] Reports of surgical correction of hallux valgus deformities date back as early as Gernet in 1836, and since then more than 130 procedures have been described.[4–7] This is no doubt a reflection of what may seem to be a simple pathology but is actually a complex 3-dimensional deformity.

Although many soft-tissue procedures have been described, metatarsal osteotomies were among the earliest techniques developed for the treatment of hallux valgus.[8] Broadly speaking, metatarsal osteotomy may be undertaken proximally or distally. Proximal osteotomy allows a greater correction than distal osteotomy,

The Foot & Ankle Unit, Department of Trauma & Orthopaedics, Barts Health NHS Trust, The Royal London Hospital, Whitechapel Road, London E1 1BB, UK
* Corresponding author.
E-mail address: fmalagelada@gmail.com

Foot Ankle Clin N Am 25 (2020) 345–359
https://doi.org/10.1016/j.fcl.2020.05.001
1083-7515/20/© 2020 Elsevier Inc. All rights reserved.

which is more commonly used for mild or moderate deformities.[8] In recent years, intermediate diaphyseal osteotomies, such as the Scarf osteotomy, have become popular.[8–10]

Within many surgical specialities, there has been an exponential growth in minimally invasive techniques. The theoretic benefits of reduced soft tissue damage, lower infection rates, preservation of vascular supply, faster rehabilitation, and being better tolerated by patients are all very appealing.

Percutaneous or minimally invasive surgery (MIS) has become increasingly popular making the results achieved in forefoot surgery comparable with the more traditional open approaches.[4,11]

The first attempts at MIS/percutaneous surgery date back to podiatric physicians in 1940s United States, attempting to bypass strict laws on surgery limiting what they could legally do.[5] However, it is widely accepted that the beginning of true minimally invasive foot surgery lies with the subcapital osteotomy technique. This was developed by Bosch's modification of the Kramer osteotomy in the 1990s, with his 7- to 10-year follow-up published in 2000.[12]

Early techniques of MIS for hallux valgus correction also included the Reverdin-Isham technique and the simple, effective, rapid, inexpensive (SERI) technique, as well as the subcapital osteotomy. However, excellent postoperative outcomes reported by the original investigators were not reproducible with the early generation techniques.

These techniques all lacked any definitive internal fixation, and one theory for the difficulties initially may well be related to lack of stability at the osteotomies. With the incorporation of internal fixation metalwork, stability could be controlled in all 3 planes of movement, and further techniques were described with excellent results.[13]

The aim of this review paper is to assess the outcomes of MIS in treating hallux valgus deformities.

METHODS

Several previous reviews on MIS hallux valgus surgery have been performed.[4,11,14–19] One of the most comprehensive reviews published to date, was a systematic review by the senior author of this paper, summarizing articles between January 2001 and January 2018.[19] The authors have extended this to now include all papers meeting the inclusion criteria up to December 2019.

The decision to select research from 2001 onward was designed to capture the newer MIS techniques developed. Studies published before 2001 reported only on the Bosch technique and during a time when MIS was not as widespread in its use, where many surgeons were at the beginning of the learning curve. Equally, given the substantial differences between some of the MIS techniques it was deemed appropriate to subdivide studies into groups to better analyze individual techniques.

Pubmed, Medline, EMBASE, Cochrane database, and Google Scholar searches were performed to identify studies. Medical subject headings terms used in the searches included and combined "hallux valgus", "bunion", "percutaneous", "minimally invasive", "MIS", "MICA", as well as specific search terms for each procedure, namely Bosch, SERI, Endolog, and Reverdin. Literature was limited to publications since 2001. Other inclusion criteria were English language publications, publications with full text, human patients treated with minimally invasive hallux valgus surgery and mean age greater than 18 years, and at least 10 patients with minimum follow-up of 1 year and reporting at least one outcome measure relating to pain or function plus radiographic evaluation and complication rates (including recurrence).

Exclusion criteria comprised any paper that did not meet the inclusion criteria, as well as those that included patients with concomitant lesser toes or other surgery of the foot and techniques that involved joint arthrodesis (ie, Lapidus, first metatarsophalangeal arthrodesis). Use of MIS procedures in revision surgery was also excluded.

As in the original review, 2 reviewers independently extracted data from each included study using a data extraction form developed for this review. Data included demographic information, methodology, details on interventions, and reported outcomes. Data were also collected on the type of scoring system used, its results, and radiological parameters, such as the hallux valgus angle (HVA) and intermetatarsal angle (IMA). A record was made of all reported complications and cases of recurrence.

Complications were subclassified as major and minor. Those considered major entail a failure to correct the deformity or complications that place a significant risk to the patient and/or affect the long-term outcome. These included recurrence, nonunion, malunion, transfer metatarsalgia, avascular necrosis, hallux varus, complex regional pain syndrome, deep infection, deep vein thrombosis, and persistent numbness-paraesthesia. Minor complications identified included K-wire issues, pin infection, delayed wound healing, metalwork failure, delayed union, superficial infection, stiffness, osteoarthritic changes, and skin burn.

RESULTS

The studies were identified by performing searches of the aforementioned databases for dates between January 2001 and December 2019. Once all papers were identified, the previous review form by the senior author of this paper was cross-referenced to ensure matching papers were selected and thus verifying the selection protocols. Between January 2018 and December 2019, thirty-six new research articles were identified that met the search criteria, of which only 5 met the inclusion criteria for this review.

In total, 328 studies were identified through the searches and only 27 studies met the inclusion criteria and were included in this systematic review.[20–46] The included studies are summarized in **Table 1**.

In total, 2577 feet in 2060 patients underwent MIS intervention across all studies included. There were 156 (7.6%) male patients across all the studies. Overall mean age was 49.67 years (12–89 years). Most of the data were level IV evidence and subsequently it was determined that further pooling of the data was not indicated. Significant methodological differences between the studies meant that there were insufficient data to perform a formal meta-analysis. These differences included indications for surgery, heterogeneity in participants, and outcome measures.

The studies were divided into categories based on the underlying principle of the surgical technique. The 5 subgroups were Bosch-type osteotomies including the SERI technique, Reverdin-type osteotomies, techniques using the Endolog prosthesis, distal soft tissue procedures, and chevron-type osteotomies.

Table 2 summarizes the radiological and patient-reported outcome measures. **Table 3** summarizes the stated complication rate in each study.

BOSCH-TYPE OSTEOTOMIES

Thirteen studies reported on Bosch or variations of this osteotomy.[20–32] In 11 reports, the procedure consisted of subcapital osteotomy of the metatarsal and temporary fixation with percutaneous K-wire. Lucattelli and colleagues[31] and Liuni and colleagues[32] used no internal fixation and maintained correction using the dressing alone.

The 13 studies reported on 1719 feet in 1295 patients, with a combined mean age of 49.4 (16–87) years and combined mean follow-up of 35.0 (12–84) months. The ranges

Table 1
Overview of included studies

Surgical Technique	Author, Year of Publication	Level of Evidence	Study Design	Number of Patients	Number of Feet	Male (%)	Age	Follow-Up
BOSCH (including SERI)	Magnan et al,[20] 2005	IV	Case series	82	118	5 (6)	56.3 ± 13 (17–79)	35.9 ± 10.9 (24–78)
	Lin et al,[21] 2009	IV	Case series	31	47	4 (13)	40.8 (13–63)	23.7 (16–68)
	Maffulli et al,[22] 2009	III	Retrospective comparative	36	36	0	51.5 ± 13.1 (21–70)	25 ± 3.2
	Siclari et al,[23] 2009	IV	Case series	49	59	5 (10)	54.6 (24–70)	31.48 (12–48)
	Enan et al,[24] 2010	IV	Case series	24	36	4 (16)	37.8 ± 12.7 (17–52)	21(12–36)
	Tong et al,[25] 2011	IV	Case series	20	23	2 (10)	55.1 (29–75)	22 (12–60)
	Radwan et al,[26] 2012	II	Prospective comparative	29	31	4 (14)	32.7 ± 7.4	21.7 (12–36)
	Scala et al,[27] 2013	IV	Case series	126	146	11 (9)	52.6 (16–87)	29.1 (12–54)
	Giannini et al,[29] 2013	II	Prospective comparative	20	20	0	53 ± 11	7 y
	Gadek et al,[28] 2013	IV	Case series	54	54	?	45.7	18
	Giannini et al,[30] 2013	IV	Case series	577	896	61 (10)	49 (20–65)	7 y (5–10)
	Liuni et al,[32] 2018	IV	Case series	52	58	3 (5%)	64 (28–82)	25 (12–48)
	Lucattelli et al,[31] 2019	IV	Retrospective case series	195	195	18(9)	49.4 (20–70)	34.6
Total/Mean				1295	1719	9% (n = 117)	49.4	35.0

	Study	Level	Study type	Patients	Feet	Complications n (%)	Age	FU
REVERDIN	Bauer et al,[33] 2009	IV	Case series	168	189	4 (2)	57 median (23–87)	13 (12–24)
	Biz et al,[34] 2016	IV	Case series	80	80	5 (7)	Median 51 ± 15.5 (26–78)	48
	Di Giorgio et al,[35] 2016[a]	II	Prospective comparative	19	19	1 (3)	23.3 ± 7.7	23.3 ± 7.7
Total/Mean				267	288	4% (n = 10)	54.5	28.1
ENDOLOG	Di Giorgio et al,[36] 2013	IV	Case series	25	33	2 (8)	52 (35–80)	18.2 (12–36)
	Biz et al,[37] 2015	IV	Case series	30	30	2 (7)	Median 56.5 (range 38–73)	48
	Di Giorgio et al,[35] 2016[a]	II	Prospective comparative	18	18	—	23.3 ± 7.7	23.3 ± 7.7
Total/Mean				73	81	7% (n = 4)	54.25	29.8
Distal Soft Tissue Release	Lui et al,[38] 2008	IV	Case series	83	94	8 (10)	45.6 (14–89)	30.45 (24–74)
	Martinez-Nova et al,[39] 2011	IV	Case series	79	79	0	54.7 ± 12.5	28.1 (24–33)
Total/Mean				162	173	5% (n = 8)	41.7	29.28
CHEVRON	Lucas Y Hernandez et al,[40] 2016	IV	Case series	38	54	3 (8)	48 (17–69)	59.1 (45.9–75.2)
	Brogan et al,[41] 2016	III	Retrospective Cohort Study	?49	49	3 (6)	53 ± 10.8	31 ± 3.5 (26–39)
	Jowett Group A,[42] 2017	IV	Case series	36	53	1 (3)	56 ± 13.1 (28–81)	26 ± 12.0 (18–38)
	Jowett Group B,[42] 2017	IV	Case series	42	53	1 (2)	54 ± 13.5 (25–77)	24 ± 5.0 (18–28)
	Lai et al,[43] 2017	III	Retrospective comparative	29	29	4 (14)	54.3 ± 12.8	24
	Holme et al,[44] 2019	IV	Case series	40	40	2 (5)	51 (18–87)	12 (12–12)
	Choi et al,[45] 2019	III	Case control	21	25	0 (0)	21.3 ± 5.1	19.9 ± 1.1
	Chan et al,[46] 2019	IV	Case series	8	13	3 (23)	50.7 (36.1–70.7)	2.9 y (2.1–3.3)
Total/Mean				263	316	6.5% (n = 17)	48.5	28.6
OVERALL				2060	2577	7.6% (n = 156)	49.67	

Abbreviation: FU, follow-up (in months, unless when stated in years).

[a] Same study by Di Giorgio et al[35] comparing 2 groups of Endolog versus Reverdin procedures.

Adapted from Malagelada F, Sahirad C, Dalmau-Pastor M, et al. Minimally invasive surgery for hallux valgus: a systematic review of current surgical techniques. Int Orthop. 2019 Mar;43(3):625–637; with permission.

Table 2
Radiographic and clinical outcomes

Procedure	Author	HVA			IMA			AOFAS		
		Pre	Post	Diff	Pre	Post	Diff	Pre	Post	Diff
BOSCH	Lin et al,[21] 2009	26 ± 4.9 (18–37)	14.2 ± 6.7 (0–26)	11.8	11.6 ± 1.6 (8–15)	5.3 ± 2.3 (0–10)	6.3	-	92.7 ± 6.2 (78–100)	-
	Maffulli et al,[22] 2009	27 ± 6	17 ± 4	10	15 ± 6	8 ± 3	7	-	-	-
	Magnan et al,[20] 2005	31.5 ± 10.2 (18–42)	13.7 ± 6.7 (7–25)	17.8	12.3 ± 3 (10–20)	7.3 ± 2.7 (4–16)	5	-	88.2 ± 12.9	-
	Siclari et al,[23] 2009	27.9 (12–45)	12.3 (2–21)	15.6	16.5 (8–25)	9.3 (3–15)	7.2	45 (30–65)	90.6 (75–100)	45.6
	Enan et al,[24] 2010	27.7 ± 3.8 (18–36.8)	14.6 ± 5.8 (8–25.4)	13.1	11.2 ± 1.8 (9.8–18)	5.8 ± 2.4 (4–11.6)	5.4	-	91.1 ± 6.8	-
	Radwan et al,[26] 2012	27.6 ± 4.4	13.1 ± 2.8	14.5	12.6 ± 2.0	7.8 ± 1.3	4.8	44.6	90.2 ± 6.8	45.6
	Scala et al,[27] 2013	32.3 ± 7.6 (12–52)	4.5 ± 5 (20 to −4)	27.8	14.4 ± 3.5 (9–22)	4.8 ± 3.4 (0–16)	9.6	54.6 ± 9.6 (12–77)	85.3 ± 18.4 (23–100)	30.7
	Giannini et al,[29] 2013	35.8 ± 3.5	21.8 ± 4.1	14	16.1 ± 3.9	6.8 ± 4.3	9.3	51 ± 10	81.2 ± 15.1	30.2
	Gadek et al,[28] 2013	33.9	14.2	19.7	14.8	9.7	5.1	37	90.7	53.7
	Giannini et al,[30] 2013	32 ± 8.3 (25–50)	13.3 ± 6.4 (4–28)	18.7	14.3 ± 3.3 (10–18)	6.9 ± 3.6 (2–14)	7.4	46.8 ± 16.7 (15–78)	89 ± 10.3 (50–100)	42.2
	Tong et al,[25] 2011	31.3 ± 5.3 (20–38)	15.7 ± 5.4 (2–24)	15.6	16.7 ± 2.8 (10–20)	7.7 ± 3.8 (4–14)	9	53	91.8 ± 7.9 (68–100)	38.8
	Liuni et al,[32] 2018	34.0 ± 9	10.6 ± 6	23.4	13.5 ± 3	8.5 ± 2	5	28.6 ± 14.1	91.7 ± 10.6	63.1
	Lucattelli et al,[31] 2019	Not documented	Not documented	15.5	Not documented	Not documented	5.4	54.7	89.6	34.9
Totals	Δ Range	Not documented	Not documented	10–23.4	Not documented	Not documented	4.8–9.6		81.2–92.7	30.2–63.1
REVERDIN	Bauer et al,[33] 2009	30 (25–32)	15 (11–18)	14	14 (12–15)	11 (9–13)	3	52 (44–60)	93 (82.5–100)	41
	Biz et al,[34] 2016	26.40 ± 0.64 (10–47.5)	13.90 ± 6.25 (0–34)	12.5	12.9 ± 2.83 (7.5–20)	9.00 ± 2.04 (5–14)	3.9	54.1 ± 8.3	87.1 ± 12.8	33.1
	Di Giorgio[35,a]	30.2 ± 6.6	13.1 ± 4.9	17.1	14.1 ± 2.2	8.9 ± 2.4	5.2	40.5	90.3	49.8
Totals	Δ Range			12.5–17.1			3–5.2		87.1–93	33.1–49.8

Technique	Study	HVA Pre	HVA Post	HVA Diff	IMA Pre	IMA Post	IMA Diff	AOFAS Pre	AOFAS Post	AOFAS Diff
ENDOLOG	Di Giorgio[36]	36.6 ± 8.1 (20–53)	22.7 ± 6.7 (8–32)	13.9	16.0 ± 1.9 (14–19.9)	6.1 ± 2.9 (3–11)	9.9	22.1 ± 11.1 (0.34)	88.2 ± 6.1 (85–100)	66.1
	Biz et al,[37] 2015	33.38 ± 10.72 (17.84–66.62)	16.57 ± 5.40 (7.18–25.18)	16.8	12.31 ± 3.05 (7.09–18.55)	6.36 ± 1.38 (7.74–4.98)	5.9	28.7 (19–42)	93.98	65.3
	Di Giorgio[35,a]	27.5 ± 7.2	13.4 ± 4.4	14.1	15.9 ± 3	8.2 ± 1.9 d	7.7	32.4	89.2	56.8
Totals	Δ Range			13.9–16.8			5.9–9.9		88.2–94	56.8–66.1
DSTR	Lui et al,[38] 2008	33 ± 7 (20–58)	14 ± 5 (4–30)	19	14 ± 3 (10–26)	9 ± 2 (5–18)	5	–	93 ± 8	
	Martinez-Nova et al,[39] 2011	24.1 ± 3.7	11 ± 1.7	13.1	11.8 ± 0.5	9.5 ± 0.5	2.3	68.5 ± 10.6	86.6 ± 8.5	18.1
Totals	Δ Range			13.1–19			2.3–5.0		86.6–93	18.1
CHEVRON	Lucas Y Hernandez et al,[40] 2016	26.2 ± 4.9 (16–40)	9.6 ± 3.1 (4–18)	16.6	11.8 ± 2.7 (6–18)	7.9 ± 2.1 (3–11)	3.9	62.5 ± 8.0 (30–80)	97.1 ± 5.4 (75–100)	34.6
	Brogan et al,[41] 2016	26.6 ± 10.6	10.4 ± 5.7	16.2	11.7 ± 4.4	6.8 ± 3.6	4.9	–	–	–
	Jowett Group A,[42] 2017	28.7 ± 8.1 (12–46)	10.6 ± 5.4 (4–25)	18.1	13.6 ± 3.3 (8–20)	8.1 ± 3.6 (3–15)	5.5	55 ± 11.3 (23–76)	85 ± 9.3 (75–98)	30
	Jowett Group B,[42] 2017	30.7 ± 5.7 (20–44)	9.9 ± 4.01 (0–18)	20.8	14.4 ± 1.8 (10–18)	7.1 ± 1.8 (4–12)	7.3	57 ± 8.6 (42–76)	89 ± 10.9 (50–100)	32
	Lai et al,[43] 2017	29.9 ± 8.5	8.8 ± 5.9	21.1	14.6 ± 3.9	10.3 ± 3.1	4.3	58.6 ± 16.6	87.4 ± 17.8	28.8
	Holme et al,[44] 2019	31.7 (12–57)	12.1 (1–43)	19.6	13.2 (6–24)	6.7 (2–13)	6.5	48.2 (24–72)	93.4 (60–100)	45.2
	Choi et al,[45] 2019	25.3 ± 3.4	12.4 ± 4.6	12.9	14.4 ± 0.8	4.9 ± 2.2	9.5	58.6 ± 8.6	88.9 ± 6.4	30.3
	Chan et al,[46] 2019	30.4 ± 5.9 (17.9–39.4)	10.9 ± 7.2 (0.55–20.8)	19.5	13.9 ± 3.5 (range 7.5–18.8)	10.2 ± 3.3 (4.9–15.2)	3.7	59.0 ± 13.1	93.7 ± 8.0	34.7
Totals	Δ Range			12.9–21.1			3.7–7.3		85–97.1	28.8–34.6

Abbreviations: Δ, difference in; AOFAS, American Orthopaedic Foot and Ankle Score; Diff, difference in value between pre- and postoperative; DSTR, distal soft tissue release; HVA, hallux valgus angle; IMA, intermetatarsal angle; Post, postoperative value; Pre, preoperative value.

a Same study by Di Giorgio et al[35] comparing 2 groups of Endolog versus Reverdin procedures.

Adapted from Malagelada F, Sahirad C, Dalmau-Pastor M, et al. Minimally invasive surgery for hallux valgus: a systematic review of current surgical techniques. Int Orthop. 2019 Mar;43(3):625-637; with permission.

Table 3
Complications

Author	Feet	Major n	%	Minor n	%	Totals n	%
BOSCH							
Lin et al,[21] 2009	47	1	2%	8	17%	9	19%
Maffulli et al,[22] 2009	36	0	0%	1	3%	1	3%
Magnan et al,[20] 2005	118	2	2%	9	8%	11	9%
Siclari et al,[23] 2009	59	4	7%	1	2%	5	8%
Enan et al,[24] 2010	36	4	11%	3	8%	7	19%
Radwan et al,[26] 2012	31	0	0%	4	13%	4	13%
Scala et al,[27] 2013	146	7	5%	6	4%	13	9%
Giannini et al,[29] 2013	20	0	0%	0	0%	0	0%
Gadek et al,[28] 2013	54	0	0%	1	2%	1	2%
Giannini et al,[30] 2013	896	67	7%	21	2%	88	10%
Tong et al,[25] 2011	23	0	0%	5	22%	5	22%
Liuni et al,[32] 2018	58	9	16%	9	16%	16	32%
Lucattelli et al,[31] 2019	195	12	6%	7	4%	19	10%
Totals	1719	106	6%	75	4%	179	10%
REVERDIN							
Bauer et al,[33] 2009	189	8	4%	2	1%	10	5%
Biz et al,[34] 2016	80	5	6%	1	1%	6	8%
Di Giorgio[a]	19	0	0%	0	0%	0	0%
Totals	288	13	5%	3	1%	16	6%
CHEVRON							
Lucas Y Hernandez et al,[40] 2016	54	0	0%	5	9%	5	9%
Brogan et al,[41] 2016	49	5	10%	4	8%	9	18%
Jowett Group A,[42] 2017	53	9	17%	12	23%	21	40%
Jowett Group B,[42] 2017	53	7	13%	7	13%	14	26%

(continued on next page)

	Feet	Major		Minor		Totals	
Author		n	%	n	%	n	%
Lai et al,[43] 2017	29	0	0%	0	0%	0	0%
Holme et al,[44] 2019	40	0	0%	4	4%	4	4%
Choi et al,[45] 2019	25	0	0%	2	8%	2	8%
Chan et al,[46] 2019	13	3	23%	2	15%	5	38%
Totals	316	24	8%	36	11%	60	19%[b]
ENDOLOG							
Di Giorgio	33	0	0%	0	0%	0	0%
Biz et al,[37] 2015	30	2	7%	1	3%	3	10%
DiGiorgio[a]	18	0	0%	0	0%	0	0%
Totals	81	2	3%	1	2%	3	4%
DSTR							
Lui et al,[38] 2008	94	3	3%	1	1%	4	4%
Martínez-Nova et al,[39] 2011	79	0	0%	0	0%	0	0%
Totals	173	3	2%	1	1%	4	2%
TOTALS	2577	148	6%	116	4%	262	10%

Table 3
(*continued*)

Abbreviation: DSTR, distal soft tissue release.

[a] Same study by Di Giorgio et al[35] comparing 2 groups of Endolog versus Reverdin procedures.

[b] The study by Jowett is the only one to include a subgroup of patients during the early stages of the learning curve of the surgeon. If this subgroup were to be excluded from the analysis the overall complication rate for the chevron Akin group would be 12% instead of 19%.

Adapted from Malagelada F, Sahirad C, Dalmau-Pastor M, et al. Minimally invasive surgery for hallux valgus: a systematic review of current surgical techniques. Int Orthop. 2019 Mar;43(3):625-637; with permission.

in improvement in HVA were 10 to 23.4°, IMA 4.8 to 9.6°, and American Orthopedic Foot and Ankle Score (AOFAS) ranging from 30.2 to 63.1. Overall complication rate was 10%.

The largest study in this subgroup was that by Gianni and colleagues.[30] Six hundred forty-one patients were prospectively studied, amounting to 896 feet at final follow-up. All patients underwent the SERI technique, with average follow-up of 7 years, with a range of 5 to 10 years. The average AOFAS significantly improved at last follow-up to an average of 89 $\pm$ 10.3, whereas preoperatively it was 46.8 $\pm$ 16.7 ($P < .001$). The mean HVA value decreased from 32° $\pm$ 8.3 preoperatively to 13.3° $\pm$ 6.4 at last follow-up ($P < .05$). The mean IMA value decreased from 14.3° $\pm$ 3.3 preoperatively to 6.9° $\pm$ 3.6 at last follow-up ($P < .05$). The mean DMAA value decreased from 13.5° $\pm$ 5.3 preoperatively to 6.5° $\pm$ 4.4 at last follow-up ($P < .05$). A complication rate of 10% was noted.

The most recent paper published was by Lucatelli and colleagues.[31] One hundred ninety-five consecutive patients with isolated symptomatic HV were surgically treated using a percutaneous technique without any form of internal fixation, with a mean follow-up of 34.6 months. The AOFAS improved from a preoperative median of 54.7 to 89.6 at 2 years follow-up ($P = .002$). Patients were satisfied or very satisfied in 94% of cases at the latest follow-up. A mean radiographic correction of the HVA of 15.5°, IMA of 5.4°, and DMAA of 5.4° was achieved. A total of 19 (9.7%) complications were reported.

REVERDIN-ISHAM

Three studies evaluated the Reverdin-Isham technique, which involves an intraarticular medial wedge closing osteotomy of the first metatarsal.[32–35] It is usually accompanied by a medial eminence resection, Akin osteotomy of the proximal phalanx, and distal soft tissue release without any form of internal fixation.

The 3 studies reported on 288 feet in 267 patients, with a combined mean age of 54.5 (23–87) years and a combined mean follow-up of 28.1 (12–48) months. The ranges in improvement in HVA were 12.5 to 17.1°, IMA 3 to 5.2°, and AOFAS 33.1 to 49.8. Overall complication rate was 5.5%.

Bauer and colleagues[33] present the largest study with 189 feet. One hundred sixty-eight consecutive subjects were included in the present prospective multicenter study. One hundred fifty-six subjects (87%) were satisfied or very satisfied with the outcome of the procedure. The median postoperative AOFAS was 93 points. Subjects averaged a loss of 17% of first metatarsophalangeal joint motion. The median HVA and IMA improved from 28° and 13° preoperatively, to 14° and 10° postoperatively, respectively.

ENDOLOG PROCEDURES

Three studies reported on the use of the Endolog device, a curved titanium partially intramedullary nail, which serves to laterally translate the metatarsal head and does not require routine removal.[35–37]

The 3 studies reported on 81 feet in 73 patients, with a combined mean age of 54.25 (35–80) years and a combined mean follow-up of 29.8 (12–48) months. The ranges of improvement in HVA were 13.9 to 16.8°, IMA 5.9 to 9.9°, and AOFAS 56.8 to 66.1. The overall complication rate was 4%.

Di Giorgio and colleagues[35] presented a comparison of the Reverdin and Endolog procedures. The Endolog group achieved an average correction of HVA and IMA of 14°±6.2° and 7.7°±2.6°, respectively. The mean AOFAS improved from a preoperative of 32.4 ± 16.8 points to 89.2 ± 10.5. No statistically significant differences were detected between the 2 groups with respect to the AOFAS score, HVA, and IMA. Both groups showed good to excellent results. No complications were noted in the Endolog group.

DISTAL SOFT TISSUE PROCEDURES

Two studies reported on a distal soft tissue release assisted by either arthroscopy or fluoroscopy. In the first study, a screw between the first and second metatarsals was introduced and in the second, an Akin osteotomy was performed under fluoroscopy.[38,39]

The 2 studies reported on 173 feet in 162 patients, with a combined mean age of 41.7 (14–89) years and a combined mean follow-up of 29.28 (12–74) months. The ranges of improvement in HVA were 13.1 to 19°, IMA 2.3 to 5.0°, and AOFAS 18.1, but only 1 of the 2 studies reported a pre- and postoperative AOFAS. The overall complication rate was 2%. It is worth mentioning that only a 2° reduction in IMA was produced in the paper describing distal soft tissue release and Akin osteotomy,[39] hence not a suitable technique for those moderate-severe corrections.

MINIMALLY INVASIVE CHEVRON AND AKIN

Seven studies reported on this MIS technique, with Jowett and Bedi[42] reporting on 2 groups including a subgroup of patients during the early stages of the learning curve of the surgeon. There were studies reporting on the percutaneous extraarticular reverse-L chevron (PERC) osteotomy, which also included an Akin osteotomy, and others on the minimally invasive chevron Akin (MICA), also called percutaneous chevron Akin (PECA). The 2 techniques differ in the use of 1 (PERC) or 2 (MICA/PECA) screws for fixation of the metatarsal osteotomy. The theory is that with the MICA/PECA procedure, higher degrees of correction can be achieved. In the PERC procedure, the screw is inserted from dorsal to plantar and in the MICA/PECA from medial to lateral.

The 7 studies reported on 316 feet in 263 patients, with a combined mean age of 48.5 (17–87) years and a combined mean follow-up of 28.6 (12–75.2) months. The ranges of improvement in HVA were 12.9 to 21.1°, IMA 3.7 to 7.3, and AOFAS 28.8 to 34.6. The overall complication rate was 19%.

Jowett and Bedi[42] presented the first MICA experience of the senior author involving 106 patients, divided into 2 groups, with the first 53 feet going into group A and the second 53 feet going into group B. Overall, the mean AOFAS improved from 56 (range 23–76) preoperatively to 87 (range 50–100) postoperatively (P<.001). The mean HVA and IMA improved from preoperative 29.7° (range 12–46°) and 14.0° (range 8–20°) to 10.3° (range 0–25°) and 7.6° (range 3–15; P<.001), respectively. Between the groups, they seemed to demonstrate a significant learning curve, with lower revision rate and higher satisfaction rate with the group B patients.

COMBINED OUTCOMES

Across the 2552 feet in 2026 patients, the mean age was 46.51 (8.1–89) years. Overall, range of improvement of HVA was 8.6 to 21.1, IMA 0.9 to 9.6, and AOFAS 18.1 to 66.1. Complication rates varied from 0% to 40%, with a mean rate of 10% (6% major complications, 4% minor complications).

DISCUSSION

MIS in the treatment of hallux valgus deformity has gained increasing popularity since the 1990s. The appeal of minimizing soft tissue damage, reducing surgical time, and faster recovery is offset by the initial learning curve and a lack of robust, high-quality evidence to support minimally invasive over open surgical techniques.

Most of the research in minimally invasive hallux valgus surgery continues to represent level IV evidence, and there is the ongoing need for further, larger randomized control trials with greater focus on patient-reported outcome measures (PROMs). Although there are numerous papers that focus on the retrospective assessment of radiological improvements after MIS procedures, there are a limited number that report pre- and postoperative PROMs. We were not able to identify any level I evidence regarding MIS hallux valgus surgery. Three of the 27 studies included were level II evidence, 4 further studies were level III evidence, and the remaining 20 studies were level IV data. Because of the heterogeneity of methodologies, patient populations, and outcomes measures, pooling the data was not possible, nor was formal meta-analysis.

Despite these issues, this review suggests that MIS hallux valgus surgery, as a whole, is a safe and effective method of treating hallux valgus deformities, with an acceptable risk profile.

As mentioned, 3 randomized control studies were included in this review.[26,29,35] The first study by Radwan and Mansour[26] compared percutaneous distal metatarsal osteotomy with open distal chevron osteotomy in 64 feet with mild to moderate hallux valgus. Thirty-one feet underwent the modified Bosch procedure and 33 underwent the open chevron. Improvements in HVA, IMA, and AOFAS were comparable between the 2 groups, but the MIS group showed faster surgical times and greater satisfaction with cosmesis. The investigators performed a power calculation to identify a sample size to identify statistically significant differences in AOFAS but not radiographic parameters or complication rates.[26]

Gianni and colleagues[29] performed a randomized control trial to determine whether SERI or Scarf osteotomy was associated with better functional outcomes, radiographic correction, and fewer complications at 2- and 7-year follow-up. Twenty patients with bilateral hallux valgus were treated one side with SERI and the other side with Scarf osteotomy. No differences were found between the 2 groups. In 2016, Di Giorgio and colleagues[35] compared Reverdin-Isham and Endolog in a total of 40 patients, 20 in each group. No significant differences were found in either group with respect to radiological markers of improvement or AOFASs. Neither of these studies document the use of a power calculation to determine sample size to identify statistically significant results.

Although not included in this review, because of failure to meet the minimum follow-up criteria, Kaufmann and colleagues[4] recently compared minimally invasive chevron with open chevron in their randomized control trial. Forty-seven cases were analyzed (25 MIS group; 22 open group). No significant differences were observed between the groups at any of the determined outcome parameters. However, patient satisfaction was better in the MIS group at the 12-week mark, a statistically significant finding.

Although the literature highly suggests comparative outcomes to open techniques, it does not enable the recommendation of one MIS technique over another. Conclusions can be drawn and eluded to, but none of these will have any statistical significance. Based on the data from this review, the MICA technique shows the greatest potential for HVA correction, with the Endolog showing greatest improvement in IMA correction and AOFAS improvement. The Reverdin showed the least potential for both HVA and IMA correction. As a medial closing wedge osteotomy, this lack of effect on IMA is understandable. It must be reiterated that these conclusions are drawn from marginal differences, with no underlying scientific basis.

Similarly, the complication profiles were extremely varied within each subgroup. The chevron subgroup had the highest averaged complication rate. However, it is worth mentioning that if the Jowett and colleagues' learning curve subgroup were excluded from the analysis, the overall complication rate for the chevron Akin group would be 12% instead of 19%, thus bringing it more in line to the other averaged complication rates. Another message can be derived from this paper: as expected there is a learning curve with MIS that leads to improved results. Some of the initial historical studies with poorer outcomes may have included this learning curve stage within the general results that may negatively skew the final outcomes and message.

Complications rates for each group were Bosch 0% to 32%, Reverdin 0% to 8%, Endolog 0% to 10%, DSTR 0% to 4%, and chevron 0% to 40%. Interpretation of these ranges is difficult because of the spread of complication rates. For example, in the Bosch group, 3 studies had complication rates less than 4% but 1 had a 32% complication rate, which will no doubt skew the mean. There was also heterogeneity in which complications were considered, for example, not all studies considered the same complications, with some of the studies with lower complication rates not including joint stiffness, which is a recognized complication in the Bosch technique for example,

Our findings are similar to those from previous reviews. Two of the most notable previous reviews were performed by Roukis[11] in 2009 and Trnka and colleagues[5] in 2013.

Roukis published the first review of MIS techniques, in which strict inclusion criteria meant that only 3 papers were included. They concluded that percutaneous surgical treatment of hallux valgus might provide structural realignment and patient satisfaction results comparable with traditional open approaches and could offer some advantages. Trnka's review identified the advantage of faster surgical times and the main disadvantage as joint stiffness, especially with the Bosch technique. Interestingly minimal stiffness is actually one of the advantages observed in the rest of MIS techniques that do not fix the osteotomy with a percutaneous wire. They also concluded that low reported complication rates must be considered with the experience of the operating center. Both reviews identified the need for more robust, methodologically sound studies.

SUMMARY

This review supports the previous data, to suggest that MIS hallux valgus techniques are a safe and effective method of correcting deformities. Evidence would suggest the presence of a significant learning curve with all MIS procedure. Radiological and clinical outcomes seem to be comparative to open procedures.

However, there is currently insufficient evidence to recommend MIS over open procedures for the correction of hallux valgus. There is currently insufficient evidence to recommend one minimally invasive technique over another. There is a continued need for prospective, randomized studies focusing on comparing minimally invasive techniques with both open techniques and other minimally invasive techniques, with further focus on patient reported outcome measures.

DISCLOSURE

The authors have nothing to disclose.

REFERENCES

1. Benvenuti F, Ferrucci L, Guralnik JM, et al. Foot pain and disability in older persons: an epidemiologic survey. J Am Geriatr Soc 1995;43(5):479–84.
2. Elton PJ, Sanderson SP. A chiropodial survey of elderly persons over 65 years in the community. Public Health 1986;100(4):219–22.
3. Nix S, Smith M, Vicenzino B. Prevalence of hallux valgus in the general population: a systematic review and meta-analysis. J Foot Ankle Res 2010;3:21–4.
4. Kaufmann G, Dammerer D, Heyenbrock F, et al. Minimally invasive versus open chevron osteotomy for hallux valgus correction: a randomized controlled trial. Int Orthop 2018;43(2):343–50.
5. Trnka HJ, Krenn S, Schuh R. Minimally invasive hallux valgus surgery: a critical review of the evidence. Int Orthop 2013;37(9):1731–5.
6. Ferrari J, Higgins JP, Prior TD. Interventions for treating hallux valgus (abducto-valgus) and bunions. Cochrane Database Syst Rev 2004;(1):CD000964.
7. Dayton P, Sedberry S, Feilmeier M. Complications of metatarsal suture techniques for bunion correction: a systematic review of the literature. J Foot Ankle Surg 2015;54:230–2.
8. Tsikopoulos K, Papaioannou P, Kitridis D, et al. Proximal versus distal metatarsal osteotomies for moderate to severe hallux valgus deformity: a systematic review and meta-analysis of clinical and radiological outcomes. Int Orthop 2018;42: 1853–63.

9. Robinson AH, Limbers JP. Modern concepts in the treatment of hallux valgus. J Bone Joint Surg Br 2005;87-B:1038–45.

10. Lee KB, Cho NY, Park HW, et al. A comparison of proximal and distal Chevron osteotomy, both with lateral soft-tissue release, for moderate to severe hallux valgus in patients undergoing simultaneous bilateral correction: a prospective randomised controlled trial. Bone Joint J 2015;97-B:202–7.

11. Roukis TS. Percutaneous and minimum incision metatarsal osteotomies: a systematic review. J Foot Ankle Surg 2009;48:380–7.

12. Bösch P, Wanke S, Legenstein R. Hallux valgus correction by the method of Bösch: a new technique with a seven-to-ten-year follow-up. Foot Ankle Clin 2000;5:485–98.

13. Vernois J, Redfern D. Percutaneous Chevron; the union of classic stable fixed approach and percutaneous technique. Fuss Sprunggelenk 2013;11:70–5.

14. Maffulli N, Longo UG, Marinozzi A, et al. Hallux valgus: effectiveness and safety of minimally invasive surgery. A systematic review. Br Med Bull 2011;9:149–67.

15. Mathavan G, Gaskell L, Pillai A, et al. Minimal invasive hallux valgus surgery: myth or magic. A systematic review. Orthop Rheumatol Open Access J 2015;1(1): 555551.

16. NICE. National Institute for Health and Clinical Excellence. Interventional procedure overview of surgical correction of hallux valgus using minimal access techniques. Interventional procedure guidance. 2010. Available at: https://www.nice.org.uk/guidance/ipg332/documents/surgical-correction-of-hallux-valgus-using-minimal-accesstechniques-overview2.

17. Caravelli S, Mosca M, Massimi S, et al. Percutaneous treatment of hallux valgus: what's the evidence? A systematic review. Musculoskelet Surg 2017;102(2): 111–7.

18. Bia A, Guerra-Pinto F, Pereira BS, et al. Percutaneous osteotomies in hallux valgus: a systematic review. J Foot Ankle Surg 2018;57:123–30.

19. Malagelada F, Sahirad C, Dalmau-Pastor M, et al. Minimally invasive surgery for hallux valgus: a systematic review of current surgical techniques. Int Orthop 2019;43(3):625–37.

20. Magnan B, Pezzè L, Rossi N, et al. Percutaneous distal metatarsal osteotomy for correction of hallux valgus. J Bone Joint Surg Am 2005;87:1191–9.

21. Lin YC, Cheng YM, Chang JK, et al. Minimally invasive distal metatarsal osteotomy for mild to moderate hallux valgus deformity. Kaohsiung J Med Sci 2009; 25(8):431–7.

22. Maffulli N, Longo UG, Oliva F, et al. Bosch osteotomy and scarf osteotomy for hallux valgus correction. Orthop Clin North Am 2009;40:515–24.

23. Siclari A, Decantis V. Arthroscopic lateral release and percutaneous distal osteotomy for hallux valgus: a preliminary report. Foot Ankle Int 2009;30:675–9.

24. Enan A, Abo-Hegy M, Seif H. Early results of distal metatarsal osteotomy through minimally invasive approach for mild-to moderate hallux valgus. Acta Orthop Belg 2010;76:526–35.

25. Tong CK, Ho YF. Use of minimally invasive distal metatarsal osteotomy for correction of hallux valgus. J Orthop Trauma Rehabili 2012;16:16–21.

26. Radwan YA, Mansour AM. Percutaneous distal metatarsal osteotomy versus distal chevron osteotomy for correction of mild-to-moderate hallux valgus deformity. Arch Orthop Trauma Surg 2012;132:1539–46.

27. Scala A, Vendettuoli D. Modified minimal incision subcapital osteotomy for hallux valgus correction. Foot Ankle Spec 2013;6:65–72.

28. Gadek A, Liszka H. Mini-invasiveMitchell-Kramer method in the operative treatment of hallux valgus deformity. Foot Ankle Int 2013;34:865–9.
29. Giannini S, Cavallo M, Faldini C, et al. The SERI distal metatarsal osteotomy and scarf osteotomy provide similar correction of hallux valgus. Clin Orthop Relat Res 2013;471:2305–11.
30. Giannini S, Faldini C, Nanni M, et al. A minimally invasive technique for surgical treatment of hallux valgus: simple, effective, rapid, inexpensive (SERI). Int Orthop 2013;37(9):1805–13.
31. Lucattelli G, Catani O, Sergio F, et al. Preliminary experience with a minimally invasive technique for hallux valgus correction with no fixation. Foot Ankle Int 2019;41(1):37–43.
32. Liuni FM, Berni L, Fontanarosa A, et al. Hallux valgus correction with a new percutaneous distal osteotomy: Surgical technique and medium term outcomes. Foot Ankle Surg 2018;26(1):39–46.
33. Bauer T, de Lavigne C, Biau D, et al. Percutaneous hallux valgus surgery: a prospective multicentre study of 189 cases. Orthop Clin North Am 2009;40:505–14.
34. Biz C, Fosser M, Dalmau-Pastor M, et al. Functional and radiographic outcomes of hallux valgus correction by mini-invasive surgery with Reverdin-Isham and Akin percutaneous osteotomies: a longitudinal prospective study with a 48-month follow-up. J Orthop Surg Res 2016;11:157.
35. Di Giorgio L, Sodano L, Touloupakis G, et al. Reverdin-Isham osteotomy versus Endolog system for correction of moderate hallux valgus deformity: a randomized controlled trial. Clin Ter 2016;167(6):e150–4.
36. Di Giorgio L, Touloupakis G, Simone S, et al. The Endolog system for moderate to severe hallux valgus. J Orthop Surg 2013;21:47–50.
37. Biz C, Corradin M, Petretta I, et al. Endolog technique for correction of hallux valgus: a prospective study of 30 patients with 4-years follow-up. J Orthop Surg Res 2015;10:102–15.
38. Lui TH, Chan KB, Chow HT, et al. Arthroscopy-assisted correction of hallux valgus deformity. Arthroscopy 2008;24:875–80.
39. Martínez-Nova A, Sánchez-Rodríguez R, Leal-Muro A, et al. Dynamic plantar pressure analysis and midterm outcomes in percutaneous correction for mild hallux valgus. J Orthop Res 2011;29:1700–6.
40. Lucas y, Hernandez J, Golanó P, et al. Treatment of moderate hallux valgus by percutaneous, extra-articular reverse-L Chevron (PERC) osteotomy. Bone Joint J 2016;98-B:365–73.
41. Brogan K, Lindisfarne E, Akehurst H, et al. Minimally invasive and open distal chevron osteotomy for mild to moderate hallux valgus. Foot Ankle Int 2016;37:1197–204.
42. Jowett CRJ, Bedi HS. Preliminary results and learning curve of the minimally invasive Chevron akin operation for hallux valgus. J Foot Ankle Surg 2017;56:445–52.
43. Lai MC, Rikhraj IS, Woo YL, et al. Clinical and radiological outcomes comparing percutaneous Chevron-Akin osteotomies vs open scarf-akin osteotomies for hallux valgus. Foot Ankle Int 2017;1. 1071100717745282.
44. Holme TJ, Sivaloganathan SS, Patel B, et al. Third-generation minimally invasive chevron akin osteotomy for hallux valgus. Foot Ankle Int 2020;41(1):50–6.
45. Choi JY, Ahn HC, Kim SH, et al. Minimally invasive surgery for young female patients with mild-to-moderate juvenile hallux valgus deformity. Foot Ankle Surg 2019;25(3):316–22.
46. Chan CX, Gan JZ, Chong HC, et al. Two year outcomes of minimally invasive hallux valgus surgery. Foot Ankle Surg 2019;25(2):119–26.

Learning Curve for Minimally Invasive Surgery and How to Minimize It

Harvinder Bedi, MBBS, MPH, FRACS[a],*,
Ben Hickey, BM, MRCS, MSc, FRCS (Tr & Orth), MD[b]

KEYWORDS

- Learning curve • Minimally invasive • Technique • Hallux valgus • Bunion

KEY POINTS

- Cadaveric training in minimally invasive surgery is critical to enable surgeons to become familiar with instruments and key parts of the procedure such as osteotomy.
- The surgeon must pay attention to the detail of positioning of the patient, the image intensifier, burr console, and theater staff.
- Procedures take longer at the start of the learning curve, so it is important that surgeons select easier cases and allocate time to perform these.
- Minimally invasive procedures can be deconstructed into 3 components: performing, displacing, and holding the osteotomy. It is important to plan all of these steps.
- Reflecting on cases performed and measurement of outcomes enables the surgeon to continually identify areas for improvement.

INTRODUCTION

There are many important components of good surgical education, including clinical judgment, communication skills, knowledge, and technical skills.[1] In the surgical specialties, good technical skills are vital.[2] Darzi and Mackay suggest that 3 components of technical performance are intraoperative judgment, knowledge (to implement the outcome of intraoperative judgment), and dexterity (pure motor aspect).[3] It is acknowledged that good technical skills do not guarantee patient safety; however, it is known that errors in technique and judgment are among leading causes for intra-operative error.[4,5]

When a new surgical procedure is being learned, it is evident that poorer clinical outcomes are often encountered. For example, in upper limb surgery, a single surgeon

[a] Department of Orthopaedic Surgery, Box Hill Hospital, 8 Arnold Street, Box Hill, Melbourne, Victoria 3128, Australia; [b] Department of Orthopaedic Surgery, Wrexham Maelor Hospital, Croesnewydd Road, Wrexham LL13 7TD, Wales
* Corresponding author.
E-mail address: hbedi@osv.com.au

Foot Ankle Clin N Am 25 (2020) 361–371
https://doi.org/10.1016/j.fcl.2020.05.002
1083-7515/20/© 2020 Elsevier Inc. All rights reserved.

series of 200 reverse total shoulder replacements revealed an early local complication rate of 23% for the first 40 cases performed in comparison to 6.5% for subsequent cases.[6] For arthroscopic or open Latarjet procedure, operative time, complication rate, and patient length of stay have all been shown to reduce with increasing surgeon experience.[7] A similar finding has been shown for lower limb arthroplasty. In a study of complications of hip resurfacing, major complications (intraoperative fracture, nerve injury, or dislocation) occurred significantly more frequently during the first 25 cases performed (28% vs 8%, $P<.002$), despite the procedures being performed by surgeons with at least 17 years in practice, who performed at least 180 total hip replacements per year.[8] Similarly, when performing total hip replacement through the direct anterior approach, a single surgeon series reported a complication rate of 44% for the first 50 cases, which reduced to 16% for the second 50 cases performed. Complication rates did not reduce to a steady state until 88 cases had been performed.[9]

For foot and ankle surgical procedures, it is also clear that a "learning curve" exists. For example, in a study of patients who underwent ankle, hindfoot, or midfoot procedures, it was shown that functional outcomes were worse for the first 27 patients performed by a new consultant in comparison to the subsequent 30 patients when measured 6 months postsurgery.[10] In the context of hallux valgus surgery, Coetzee reported a complication rate of greater than 35% in his first 20 patients who underwent open Scarf osteotomy, with only 53% of patients being satisfied at 12 months after surgery.[11] Even when the open Scarf osteotomy is performed by surgeons with experience of other open osteotomies of the first metatarsal, a technical complication occurred in 10% of 78 patients (including intraoperative fracture, failure of fixation, and screw prominence).[12] Although minimally invasive (MI) hallux valgus correction is technically challenging, it has also been shown that complications requiring further surgery reduce from 26% to 15% after the first 50 cases have been performed.[13]

The aim of this article is to discuss some key aspects of performing MI foot surgery, with specific focus on technique and intraoperative decision-making in order to minimize complications and shorten the learning curve.

EQUIPMENT

A key step in minimizing a learning curve is to become familiar with the equipment necessary to perform a procedure. MI procedures require the use of specialized equipments including burrs, hand piece, foot controller, and a burr console used in a high-torque and low-speed setting to allow tactile feedback and minimize thermal damage (**Fig. 1**A). In addition, instruments including periosteal elevators, rasp, and beaver blades are used (**Fig. 1**B). Regarding the burrs, a variety are available and it is essential that the surgeon is aware of which style of burr is best used to achieve the desired task (bump removal or osteotomy). Different sizes are also available and **Fig. 1**C illustrates the sizes used to cut different bones of the forefoot. Similarly, theater staff also require an understanding of when different forms of equipment are required and how they are put together and subsequently used. A short-term investment in them provides long-term returns. Finally, imaging and particularly the use of the mini image intensifier (I/I) has become an integral part of MI procedures. This has the advantages over standard image intensification of reduced radiation dose transfer to surgeon, staff, and patient as well as being easier to maneuver by the surgeon.

PREOPERATIVE TRAINING

Historically, technical skills have been learned using the apprenticeship model, "see one, do one, teach one," whereby a novice worked under the supervision of an

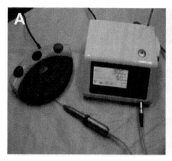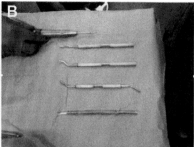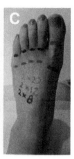

Fig. 1. (*A*) Burr Console, foot pedal, and hand piece with burr loaded. (*B*) Minimally invasive instruments including (top to bottom) hand piece and burr, straight periosteal elevator, curved periosteal elevator, dual-ended bone rasp and loaded beaver blade (*C*) Burr sizes required to create osteotomies in different bones of the forefoot.

experienced surgeon until they could independently perform operative procedures.[14] The fundamental belief in the apprenticeship model is that technical skills learned in one setting would enable performance of these skills in different settings, that is, skill transfer. Over the last decade, major changes in patient expectations, surgical practice, and working patterns have necessitated changes to the way technical skills are learned and many have suggested that allowing a novice to practice technical skills on live patients in theater for the first time is no longer appropriate.[15] As a result, the use of cadaveric training and simulation for learning technical surgical skills has emerged and has several advantages over the traditional apprenticeship model. In this context the simulation-based training allows the learner to practice their skills in a safe environment, so a higher level of competence can be attained before performance of these procedures on patients.[16,17]

Recently, well-structured simulation-based training courses have been shown to reduce perioperative complication rates for patients operated on by trainees.[18] An important part of this training is to focus on deliberate practice of focused tasks to a level of proficiency before progression to the next stage of training.[19] It is apparent that fellowship training translates to improved patient outcomes. It has recently been shown that surgeons who have completed a fellowship in arthroplasty or trauma have a lower complication rate when performing hip hemiarthroplasty when compared with those who completed a general fellowship in orthopedics.[20] For these reasons, the authors believe that appropriate training is essential in creating good outcomes and that it is poor surgical practice on the part of both the surgeon and orthopedic implant company to move straight to using MI techniques immediately on patients. This is ideally in the form of formal fellowship but for most, this lengthy pathway is unrealistic. It can also be achieved through other means including sawbone workshops, cadaver laboratories, and by observing more experienced colleagues.

Sawbone workshops provide an appreciation of the feel and sound of the burr as it cuts as well as an understanding of the movement that the surgeon's hand must make in order to achieve a correctly performed osteotomy (**Fig. 2**). Considering MI chevron and Akin osteotomy, key skills that can be practised include the metatarsal osteotomy and guidewire placement, which can be performed repetitively until confident that they can do this in the operating theater.

Cadaveric workshops provide a natural progression from sawbones to a more realistic simulation of the operative environment. The learner can link the technical steps of the procedure acquired from sawbones or similar simulation to perform the entire

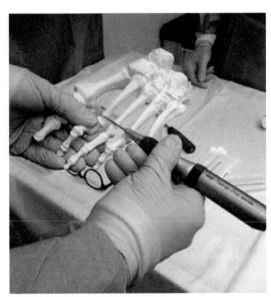

Fig. 2. Sawbone simulation showing the position of the hand after completion of a distal metatarsal minimally invasive osteotomy (DMMO).

procedure. The authors also believe that the subsequent dissection of the specimens by participants forms an important part of the learning process, as it provides immediate feedback on the performance of the desired task (eg, osteotomy) as well as information regarding the proximity of endangered structures.

Finally, direct observation with a surgeon experienced in these techniques is recommended and an opportunity taken to obtain photos of important parts of these procedures.

SET UP

A consistent and reproducible routine is required. A suggested set up is presented in **Fig. 3**. The following features should be noted. For the right hand dominant surgeon performing forefoot procedures, the authors recommend that the I/I is always brought in from the right side of the patient and that the burr console is placed on the left. Similarly, the assistant also remains on the same side as the I/I. A left-handed surgeon may choose to reverse the positioning of the equipment and assistant.

The position of the surgeon and scrub nurse usually varies according to the side that is being operated. For right foot procedures, the right-handed surgeon remains at the foot of the bed, whereas the scrub nurse moves to the patient's left. For left foot procedures, the surgeon moves to the left side and the scrub nurse to the foot of the operating table. One potential exception is that for left-sided metatarsal osteotomies, the surgeon may prefer to remain at the foot of the bed and scrub nurse to the left of the patient.

When performing a hindfoot procedure (eg, calcaneal osteotomy), the left side is performed in an unchanged fashion (ie, surgeon to the left and scrub nurse at the end of the bed). For a right-sided procedure, the surgeon moves to the right side and the assistant to the left. The scrub nurse remains at the foot of the operating table. Regarding patient positioning, the heels hang freely off the end of the operating table

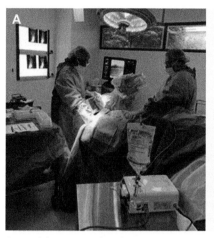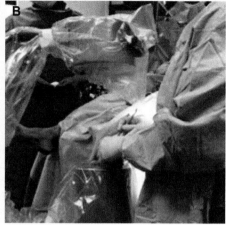

Fig. 3. (*A*) Positioning of equipment and staff during a right forefoot procedure. (*B*) Positioning of equipment and staff during a left forefoot procedure.

(**Fig. 4**). This allows easy access with the I/I as well free movement of surgeon and scrub nurse around the patient's feet.

SELECTION OF CASES

Several MI procedures have been described and each has varying degrees of difficulty. This in turn means that the number of cases taken to achieve proficiency may also vary. On occasion, the complexity of procedures may overburden the learner's attentional resources in the early stages of learning technical skills. A simple analogy is of the trainee learning to suture for the first time who uses all their attentional resources for this task and does not have any resources available for learning other aspects of the procedure. It is therefore sensible to begin with simpler procedures that have been shown to have short learning curves with low morbidity. An excellent example is of calcaneal osteotomy where high efficacy (in terms of displacement) and low morbidity have been demonstrated in relatively

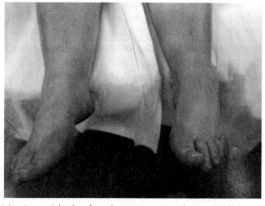

Fig. 4. Patient positioning with the feet hanging over the end of the operating table.

inexperienced hands in both cadaveric and clinical settings.[21–23] Other relatively simple procedures include distal metatarsal MI osteotomy (DMMO) and bone spur or bump resection and can also be used by the relative novice. Gradual progression should then occur to other techniques described in this journal once familiar with these simpler surgeries.

It is important to stress at this point that the indications for a particular procedure are no different to those for open surgery. It is only the technique that is different, and care must always be taken to ensure that this rule is not violated—in essence, a smaller hammer is being used to hit the same nail rather than a new hammer looking for a new nail to hit. Finally, learning new technical skills also takes extra time, a commodity that is often not readily available in the operating theater with constantly rising running costs.[24] It is essential to recognize that greater mental energy is required to perform any new procedure without adding the additional stress of an unrealistic time constraint and to organize operating list allocation accordingly. Otherwise, any opportunity for well-structured intraoperative decision-making may be compromised.

SPECIFIC TECHNICAL TIPS

All MI osteotomies have 3 key components: the cutting of the osteotomy with a burr, the displacement of the osteotomy to the desired position, and finally, the maintenance of the osteotomy (generally with screw fixation) in the desired position.

Cutting the Osteotomy

Because MI techniques use stab incisions, the use of direct vision is no longer possible and the use of other senses must compensate. Tactile feedback and sound become important sources of information for the surgeon. When the cutting portion of the burr is against or inside bone, there is a high-pitched chatter and vibration that can be felt. When in soft tissue, these are absent. It is important that this difference is recognized and should be appreciated during training sessions, as rotation of the burr in soft tissue may produce unnecessary damage and morbidity.

The use of the burr to cut the osteotomy also requires a rotational rather translational movement of the burr. The latter tends to result in stretching of the portal and consequent thermal damage as the burr rotates on the stretched skin. In order to minimize translational movement, the pivot point around which the burr is moved should therefore be at the skin surface. On occasion, it may not be possible to complete the osteotomy without stretching the portal. When this occurs, the portal may require lengthening or the hand that does not hold the burr may be used to push the skin in the same direction as the burr to reduce tension. In order to achieve this, it is important to picture the position in which the handpiece will be positioned at the beginning and end of the osteotomy. For example, when performing a DMMO, the hand piece and burr are initially positioned beside the metatarsal neck at an angle of 45° and then rotated 90° before coming to rest on top of the fifth metatarsal head (see **Fig. 2**).

Displacement of the Osteotomy

Various techniques have been described to achieve displacement of the different osteotomies to their desired positions. Before beginning the procedure, the surgeon should be aware of the most appropriate method and determine the most effective way for the assistant and scrub nurse to best assist with this. A simple example is the calcaneal osteotomy. After creation of the osteotomy, a Howarth elevator is introduced through the portal into the distal fragment and acts as a lever to displace the posterior fragment (**Fig. 5**). A more complex example is the metatarsal

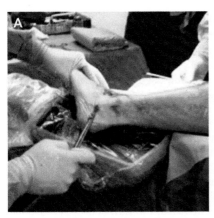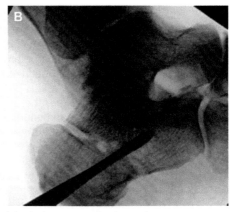

Fig. 5. (*A*) Performing calcaneal osteotomy. (*B*) Displacement of calcaneal osteotomy.

component of the MI chevron Akin osteotomy. In this case, the guidewire used for insertion of the cannulated screw was inserted into the lateral cortex before creation of the osteotomy (**Fig. 6**A), and this allows the assistant to be used (if needed) to insert the wire into a precise position while the osteotomy is held reduced by the surgeon. Displacement is achieved through the use of the periosteal elevator inserted through the osteotomy portal and used to push the capital fragment laterally. During displacement, there is a tendency for the distal fragment to flex and rotate into valgus. This is prevented by careful positioning of the surgeon's hand—the great toe is pulled against the elevator to avoid valgus angulation and the thumb placed under the metatarsal head to avoid flexion (**Fig. 6**B). Once again, these more complex maneuvers should be practiced in the workshop setting before embarking on their usage in the clinical setting.

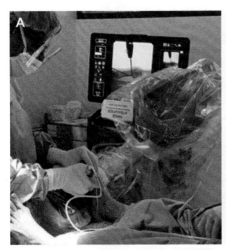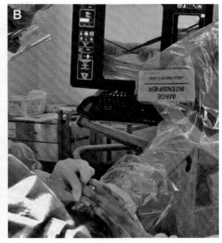

Fig. 6. (*A*) First metatarsal osteotomy. Note that this has been performed after insertion of the guidewire. (*B*) Displacement of first metatarsal osteotomy. Note the position of the surgeon's hand to avoid unwanted valgus and flexion angulation of the capital fragment.

Holding the Osteotomy

Osteotomies are generally maintained in position in 2 ways. The first is by appropriate bandaging that is typically used following claw toe correction with soft tissue release of the proximal interphalangeal joint and proximal phalangeal osteotomy. The other is the use of screws for more rigid fixation such as that used to maintain correction of metatarsal osteotomies in hallux valgus procedures.

When screw fixation is required, the use of drill guides has been very useful in limiting the skin and soft tissue damage that can often occur as both drill and screw pass through small incisions. The authors typically use a double-ended drill guide (3.2 and 4.5 mm) that will easily allow a drill and 4-mm screw to be inserted (**Fig. 7**).

A further difficulty that was previously frequently encountered was the need for metalware removal following MICA procedures. In the authors' previously published series, the rate of prominent screw removal was 13% in the first 53 cases of MI chevron and Akin, reducing to 4% for subsequent cases.[13] In view of this, it is essential to perform an intraoperative radiography in the long axis of the screw (receiver plate of the I/I parallel to the guidewire), to identify any residual protrusion of the screw head (**Fig. 8**). An additional advance seems to be the use of oblique-headed screws that are larger and therefore provide greater rigidity while avoiding this issue of prominence (**Fig. 9**).

Portal Management

The key to avoiding skin damage is by adhering to the described principles of good burr technique. Additional measures include the use of irrigation to minimize the temperature of the burr. This can be provided manually by the assistant or by the use of a burr console system that incorporates concurrent irrigation when the burr is in use (see **Fig. 3**A). If the portal is burnt or damaged, it is best to excise the damaged edges and insert a suture. Failing to do so may result in blistering or residual ooze from the portal site and an increased risk of infection. Before applying bandages it is also worthwhile

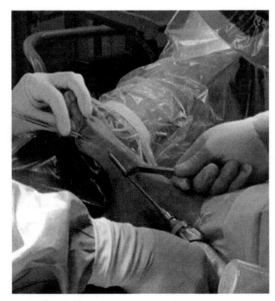

Fig. 7. Use of drill guide for drill and subsequent screw insertion.

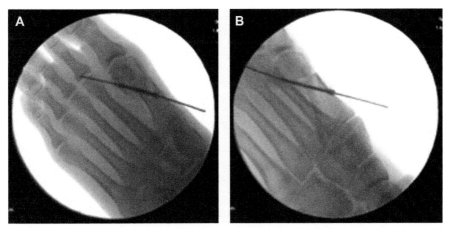

Fig. 8. (*A*) Anteroposterior image of the foot. This gives the impression that the screw is sufficiently buried. (*B*) Oblique image taken tangential to the head of the screw. This shows that the screw has poor grip on the cortex and remains prominent.

expressing any residual bone debris that may have been created at the site of any osteotomy. Manual irrigation using saline inserted through a blunt needle is also very worthwhile, as these measures will reduce the risk of heterotopic bone formation below the portal surface.

SELF APPRAISAL AND ASSESSMENT OF OUTCOMES

Finally, with all procedures, it is important to measure outcomes. This is particularly true of those that are new to the surgeon. An audit of patient satisfaction and complication rates helps to identify difficulties and allows the surgeon to modify their technique when necessary. In their study, the authors felt the screw removal rate was

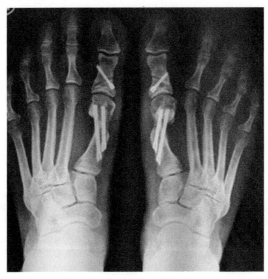

Fig. 9. Metatarsal osteotomies fixed with 4-mm oblique-headed screws.

high during the early part of the learning curve and by focusing on this as an area for improvement they were able to improve outcomes for subsequent patients.[13] This process of self-appraisal is important not only in shortening the learning curve for the surgeon themselves but also in reducing it for those in the future.

DISCLOSURE

H. Bedi is a design consultant for a company (CAB Medical) that distributes burrs and implants used in minimally invasive foot surgery.

REFERENCES

1. Thomas W. Teaching and assessing surgical competence. Ann R Coll Surg Engl 2006;88(5):429–32.
2. Gallagher AG, Ritter EM, Champion H, et al. Virtual reality simulation for the operating room. Ann Surg 2005;241(2):364–72.
3. Darzi A, Mackay S. Assessment of surgical competence. Qual Health Care 2001;(Suppl 2):ii64–9.
4. Bell RH, Biester TW, Tabuenca A, et al. Operative experience of residents in US general surgery programs: A gap between expectation and experience. Ann Surg 2009;249:719–24.
5. Fabri PJ, Zayas-Castro JL. Human error, not communication and systems, underlies surgical complications. Surgery 2008;144:557–63.
6. Kempton LB, Ankerson E, Michael Wiater J. A complication-based learning curve from 200 reverse shoulder arthroplasties. Clin Orthop Relat Res 2011;469(9): 2496–504.
7. Ekhtiari S, Horner NS, Bedi A, et al. The learning curve for the latarjet procedure: a systematic review. Orthop J Sports Med 2018;6(7):1–7.
8. Nunley RM, Zhu J, Brooks PJ, et al. The learning curve for adopting hip resurfacing among hip specialists. Clin Orthop Relat Res 2010;468(2):382–91.
9. Kong X, Grau L, Ong A, et al. Adopting the direct anterior approach: experience and learning curve in a Chinese patient population. J Orthop Surg Res 2019; 14(1):1–7.
10. Walton R, Theodorides A, Molloy A, et al. Is there a learning curve in foot and ankle surgery? Foot Ankle Surg 2012;18(1):62–5.
11. Coetzee JC. Scarf osteotomy for hallux valgus repair: the dark side. Foot Ankle Int 2003;24(1):29–33.
12. Samaras D, Gougoulias N, Varitimidis S, et al. Midterm experience of Scarf osteotomy as a new technique in a General Orthopaedic Department. Foot 2019; 40:68–75.
13. Jowett CRJ, Bedi HS. Preliminary results and learning curve of the minimally invasive chevron akin operation for hallux valgus. J Foot Ankle Surg 2017;56(3): 445–52.
14. Wigton R. See one, do one, teach one. Acad Med 1992;67(11):e45–6.
15. Leach D. In Search of Coherence: A View From the Accreditation Council for Graduate Medical Education. J Contin Educ Health Prof 2005;25(3):162–7.
16. Davies J, Aitkenhead A. Clinical risk management in anaesthesia. Clinical risk management; enhancing patient safety. 2nd edition. London: BMJ Books.; 2001.
17. Maran NJ, Glavin RJ. Low- to high-fidelity simulation - A continuum of medical education? Med Educ Suppl 2003;37:22–8.

18. Köckerling F. What is the influence of simulation-based training courses, the learning curve, supervision, and surgeon volume on the outcome in hernia repair?—a systematic review. Front Surg 2018;5:57.
19. De Win G, Van Bruwaene S, Kulkarni J, et al. An evidence-based laparoscopic simulation curriculum shortens the clinical learning curve and reduces surgical adverse events. Adv Med Educ Pract 2016;7:357–70.
20. Mabry SE, Cichos KH, McMurtrie JT, et al. Does surgeon fellowship training influence outcomes in hemiarthroplasty for femoral neck fracture? J Arthroplasty 2019;34(9):1980–6.
21. Didomenico LA, Anain J, Wargo-Dorsey M. Assessment of medial and lateral neurovascular structures after percutaneous posterior calcaneal displacement osteotomy: a cadaver study. J Foot Ankle Surg 2011;50:668.
22. Kheir E, Borse V, Sharpe J, et al. Medial displacement calcaneal osteotomy using minimally invasive technique. Foot Ankle Int 2015;36:248.
23. Jowett CRJ, Rodda D, Amin A, et al. Minimally invasive calcaneal osteotomy: A cadaveric and clinical evaluation. Foot Ankle Surg 2016;22(4):244–7.
24. Fried GM, Feldman LS, Vassiliou MC, et al. Proving the value of simulation in laparoscopic surgery. Ann Surg 2004;240:518–28.

Percutaneous Lateral Release in Hallux Valgus

Anatomic Basis and Indications

Jorge Javier Del Vecchio, MD, MBA[a,b,c],
Miki Dalmau-Pastor, PhD[a,d],*

KEYWORDS

- Hallux valgus • Percutaneous • Lateral release • Anatomic basis • Indications

KEY POINTS

- The main indications for a lateral release are mild to severe hallux valgus.
- Several studies have failed to describe accurately which structures were being released or detached as soft tissue adjuvant treatments of hallux valgus.
- Adductor tendon percutaneous release was the most commonly used procedure in order to assist osteotomies in correcting hallux valgus deformities.
- Minimally invasive surgery has an extensive learning curve and therefore it may be difficult to reproduce the results shown on published open surgery data.
- Specific cadaveric training is mandatory for any surgeon considering performing percutaneous procedures.

INTRODUCTION

Hallux valgus (HV) is a common deformity affecting the first toe, and soft tissue structures around the first metatarsophalangeal (MTP) joint are thought to play a role in its cause.[1] For this reason, the tenotomy of the adductor tendon in isolation or together

[a] GRECMIP - MIFAS (Groupe de Recherche et d'Etude en Chirurgie Mini-Invasive du Pied - Minimally Invasive Foot and Ankle Society), Merignac, France; [b] Head Foot and Ankle Section, Orthopaedics Department, Fundación Favaloro -Hospital Universitario, Solis 461, Ciudad Autónoma de Buenos Aires (CABA) CP 1078, Argentine; [c] Department of Kinesiology and Physiatry, Universidad Favaloro, Av. Entre Ríos 495, CABA CP 1079, Argentina; [d] Human Anatomy Unit, Department of Pathology and Experimental Therapeutics, School of Medicine, University of Barcelona. C/ Feixa Llarga, s/n, 08907, L'Hospitalet de Llobregat, Office 5304, Barcelona, Spain
* Corresponding author. Human Anatomy Unit, Department of Pathology and Experimental Therapeutics, School of Medicine, University of Barcelona. C/ Feixa Llarga, s/n, 08907, L'Hospitalet de Llobregat, Office 5304, Barcelona, Spain
E-mail address: mikeldalmau@ub.edu

Foot Ankle Clin N Am 25 (2020) 373–383
https://doi.org/10.1016/j.fcl.2020.05.003
1083-7515/20/© 2020 Elsevier Inc. All rights reserved.
foot.theclinics.com

with other lateral structures of the first MTP joint (lateral release) has commonly been used as an adjuvant procedure in HV surgical treatment.

Foot surgery, as with surgery in other regions, is evolving toward minimally invasive approaches, either arthroscopy or percutaneous surgery. Likewise, the adductor tenotomy or lateral release has been described as a percutaneous technique.[2–24]

In this article, an overview of the anatomy of the first MTP joint is provided, as well as a review of the supposed contributions of each structure on HV deformity. In addition, the indications of the lateral release and the different percutaneous techniques described are summarized.

Anatomy of the First Metatarsophalangeal Joint

The MTP joint of the first toe is a condyloid joint between the concave proximal surface of the proximal phalanx and the rounded head of the first metatarsal. Total range of motion of this joint is 110°, ranging from 35° plantarflexion to 75° dorsiflexion.[25]

The first MTP joint differs from the lesser toes in its bigger size and in its sesamoid mechanism,[26] embedded in the first MTP joint plantar plate. The existence of this plantar plate and its associated sesamoids is necessary because of the inherent instability of the first MTP joint, because the proximal phalanx has a shallow cavity in which the metatarsal head articulates. Most of the stability of this joint is provided by the capsular ligamentous sesamoid complex.[27] This capsular ligamentous complex is formed by a confluence of structures that includes the collateral ligaments and plantar plate, the abductor hallucis, adductor hallucis, and flexor hallucis brevis muscles.[27,28]

Thus, the joint capsule is reinforced on the plantar surface by the plantar plate, a fibrocartilaginous structure that contains the 2 sesamoid bones. The sesamoid bones, 1 medial and 1 lateral, are separated by a rounded ridge (crista) situated in the plantar articular surface of the metatarsal head, and by a fibrous groove that complements the crista (**Fig. 1**). The 2 sesamoids protrude minimally through the dorsal surface of the plantar plate, each concave longitudinally and dorsally to fit the plantar articulating surface of the metatarsal head. These sesamoids bones, compared with coffee beans by Heubach,[29] are not equal in size: the medial sesamoid is larger and longer than the

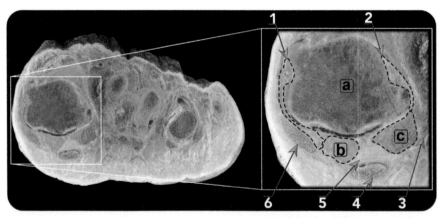

Fig. 1. Frontal cross-section of the forefoot, where the first metatarsal head (a) and the medial (b) and lateral (c) sesamoids can be observed. A mild hallux valgus deformity was present on the specimen; therefore, the metatarsal head is displaced medially. (1) Medial suspensory ligament; (2) lateral suspensory ligament; (3) adductor hallucis tendon; (4) flexor hallucis longus tendon; (5) intersesamoid ligament; (6) abductor hallucis tendon.

lateral sesamoid and tends to rest more distally. In addition to being larger, the medial sesamoid often is situated more directly under the metatarsal head, thus sustaining greater weight-bearing forces. They typically ossify between the ages of 9 and 11 years,[27] and their primary function is to dissipate force at the MTP joint and to provide mechanical advantage for the flexor hallucis brevis by elevating the metatarsal head. In addition, the sesamoids help protect the flexor hallucis longus and maintain its course along the plantar aspect of the toe.

The plantar plate of the first MTP joint is a dense mass of fibrous tissue. Its distal margin is firmly attached to the base of the phalanx, and its lateral margins receive ligamentous and muscular attachments. The proximal border receives a part of the flexor hallucis brevis before the sesamoid ligaments attach via a few loose fibers to the distal end of the metatarsal.

The medial and collateral ligaments are fan-shaped structures divided in a MTP and a metatarsosesamoid fascicle (or suspensory ligament). They are covered by the extensor sling, an aponeurotic structure that holds the extensor tendons in the right position (**Fig. 2**). Both fascicles have a common origin situated at the medial and lateral epicondyle of the metatarsal head, connected by intermediate fibers and reinforcing the joint capsule (**Fig. 3**).[26,28] The collateral ligaments fan out distally and plantarward to anchor into the base of the proximal phalanx. Their function is to provide stability to the MTP joint. The metatarsosesamoid ligaments, posterior to the collateral ones, insert into the margins of the plantar plate and their respective sesamoids (**Fig. 4**). Their function is to hold the sesamoids in their respective positions. In addition, the sesamoids are connected by the intersesamoid ligament.

The FHB divides into medial and lateral tendons that envelop the medial and lateral sesamoids. At the level of the sesamoids, the abductor hallucis tendon conjoins with the medial head of the FHB tendon, and the adductor hallucis longus conjoins with the

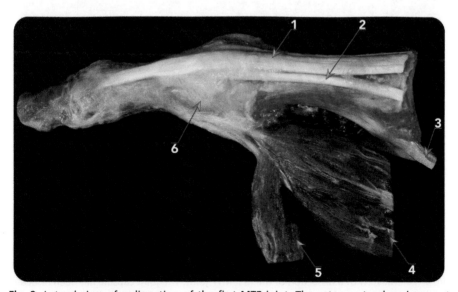

Fig. 2. Lateral view of a dissection of the first MTP joint. The extensor tendons have not been resected to show the relation between the extensor sling and the lateral collateral ligament. (1) Extensor hallucis longus tendon; (2) extensor hallucis brevis tendon; (3) peroneus longus tendon; (4) oblique head of adductor hallucis muscle; (5) transverse head of adductor hallucis muscle; (6) extensor sling.

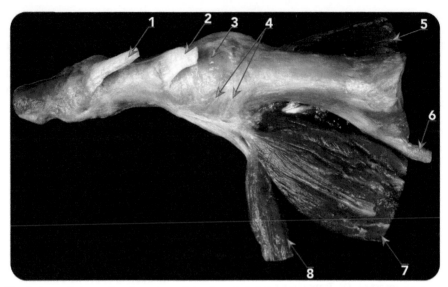

Fig. 3. Lateral view of a dissection of the first MTP joint. The extensor tendons have been resected, which allows visualization of the relation between the joint capsule and the lateral collateral ligament. (1) Extensor hallucis longus; (2) extensor hallucis brevis; (3) joint capsule; (4) lateral collateral ligament (MTP and metatarsosesamoid fascicles); (5) lateral head of flexor hallucis brevis; (6) peroneus longus tendon; (7) oblique head of adductor hallucis muscle; (8) transverse head of adductor hallucis muscle.

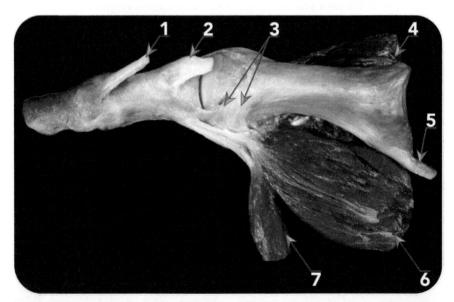

Fig. 4. Lateral view of a dissection of the first MTP joint. The joint capsule has been resected to allow visualization of the lateral collateral ligament and adductor hallucis tendon insertion. (1) Extensor hallucis longus; (2) extensor hallucis brevis; (3) lateral collateral ligament (MTP and metatarsosesamoid fascicles); (4) lateral head of flexor hallucis brevis; (5) peroneus longus tendon; (6); oblique head of adductor hallucis muscle; (7) transverse head of adductor hallucis muscle.

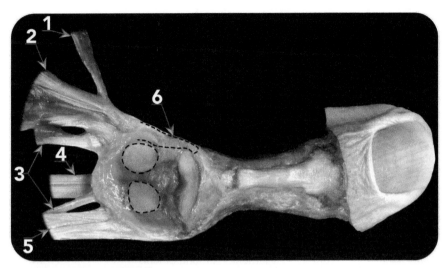

Fig. 5. Dorsal view of a dissection of the first MTP joint plantar plate. The first metatarsal has been resected. (1) Transverse head of adductor hallucis muscle; (2) oblique head of adductor hallucis muscle; (3) medial and lateral heads of flexor hallucis brevis; (4) flexor hallucis longus tendon; (5) abductor hallucis tendon; (6) area lateral to the lateral sesamoid where the percutaneous lateral release is performed.

lateral head of the FHB tendon. The FHB tendons then insert at the base of the proximal phalanx with the thick plantar plate as part of the capsular ligamentous complex. It is precisely at the area just lateral to the lateral sesamoid where the zone for the percutaneous lateral release is found (**Fig. 5**). The conjoint adductor tendon inserts in the base of the proximal phalanx, just lateral to the insertion of the plantar plate (and the phalanx-sesamoid ligament).

The capsular ligamentous sesamoid complex is fundamental during weight bearing. It must bear 40% to 60% of body weight during normal weight,[30] and peaks of force may reach 8 times body weight during running and jumping.[31]

Implications in Hallux Valgus Deformity

In an HV deformity, the adductor tendon is considered to be a deforming force on the first MTP joint, and, through its attachment on the lateral part of the base of the proximal phalanx of the first toe, it drives it into a valgus position.[26] In addition, in HV deformity, the medial displacement of the first metatarsal head causes the lateral sesamoid to be displaced off the metatarsal head. In part, this is thought to be produced by its attachment to the suspensory ligament.

Thus, resection of the adductor tendon, of the suspensory ligament of the lateral sesamoid, and even release of the conjoint tendon of flexor hallucis brevis from the lateral part of the lateral sesamoid have been described to help in restoring the first toe to its normal position.[3–6]

If HV is treated by means of percutaneous surgery, then soft tissue correction is performed through a percutaneous approach too. Numerous percutaneous techniques for the treatment of HV been described, and the use of lateral release differs among them, as do the structures claimed to be released. For some percutaneous procedures, lateral release seems not to be necessary.[32–36] However, in cases where it is included in the percutaneous HV procedure, reports in the literature may not specify which structures are released,[2,7–9] Cases where only the adductor tendon and a partial lateral capsule release is performed,[3,10–13] only the lateral suspensory ligament without affecting the adductor tendon,[6] other publications confuse the adductor and the abductor tendon[14–16] and some other variations of lateral release.[4,5,17–24]

Basic Indications of Lateral Release

The main indication for a lateral release is mild to severe HV. The combination of osteotomies and soft tissue procedures is thought to better reduce sesamoids in their anatomic position and to maintain a long-term correction when treating HV deformity.[37–39] Despite this affirmation, several studies failed to describe accurately which structures are being released or must be detached as a soft tissue adjuvant treatment of HV.[2,7–9] This fact, added to others, may explain the persistent high average overall rate of recurrence of HV deformity (4.9%).[40,41] Although both issues are difficult to address, in order to answer the first topic, some investigators mentioned that they release 1 or more of the following structures: adductor hallucis tendon,[17,19,42] adductor hallucis tendon plus partial lateral capsule release (in these cases it is not clear whether the lateral collateral ligament is included in addition to the portion of capsule released),[43] suspensory ligament,[44] among others.

There is some controversy about whether a lateral release should be performed when performing an open chevron osteotomy. Some investigators showed better results with the addition of lateral release compared with procedures without it.[45,46]

There are 2 paths to decide whether to perform a lateral release or not. One is to observe a subluxated (noncongruent) MTP joint on a weight-bearing anteroposterior radiograph. The other way is to perform a varus stress maneuver,[47] which, when positive (no MTP joint reduction) indicates that a lateral release must be performed. According to the authors, the purpose is to evaluate the true potential intermetatarsal angle. According to other investigators, this maneuver allows the surgeon to determine the displacement necessary to correct the deformity (complete sesamoid coverage).[48]

Despite this, controversy exists regarding this subject, mainly because of the lack of comparative studies and the confusion in the terminology used. Also, according to some investigators, there is a thin line between sufficient and excessive release, and the consequent risk of secondary varus deformity.[49]

The perioperative diagnosis of lateral release is challenging, particularly when minimally invasive surgery is performed because there is no direct exposure of the structures the surgeon is acting on. Surgeons need to have some indirect sign that helps to predict which structures are being released. To date, there are no studies that include radiographic proofs when doing different lateral release procedures.

Indications of Lateral Release in Relation to Severity of the Hallux Valgus Deformity

Mild deformity
An isolated adductor tendon release,[17,18] or one associated with lateral capsule percutaneous release, seems to be a frequent choice of procedure in order to correct a mild HV deformity.[3,11,50]

Moderate
Although an accurate adductor tendon and lateral capsule release may correct a congruent and incongruent moderate deformity,[3,10,14,15,22,43] some investigators included existing adherences between the lateral sesamoid bone and the plantar side of the lateral capsule to correct this type of HV.[5]

Severe

According to some investigators, it seems sufficient to release the adductor tendon and lateral capsule. This issue can be explained by the displacement power of the osteotomies used.[43,51] Other investigators prefer the addition of the release of other structures, such as the sesamoid suspensory ligament.[19]

Types of Lateral Release

Two types of lateral release exist: isolated adductor tenotomy and combined percutaneous lateral release.

Adductor release

The complete adductor tendon lateral release option may include one of these structures: partial or complete lateral capsule and lateral collateral ligament and/or suspensory ligament.

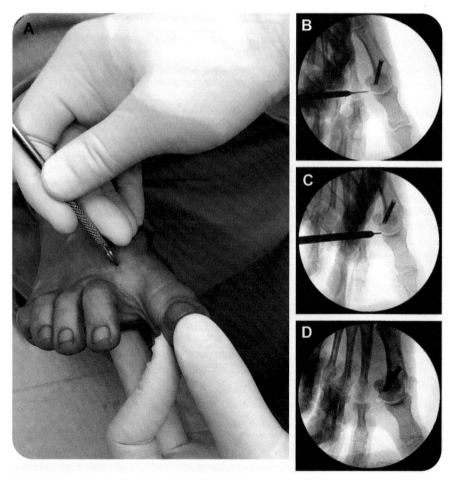

Fig. 6. Percutaneous adductor tendon release. (*A*) Incision on the first web space; (*B*) Blade progressed with 45° to 60° orientation; (*C*) less than a quarter of the blade is inside the joint; (*D*) after release of the tendon.

Combined side release

An extended version can be used in cases of moderate to severe deformity. In a recent meta-analysis, Yammine and Assi[39] concluded that there might be a beneficial effect of lateral soft tissue release (including lateral capsule of the first MTP joint, the sesamoid suspensory ligament or lateral sesamoid metatarsal ligament, and the transverse metatarsal ligament) in all cases of HV deformity, and a probable efficacy of an added adductor hallucis tendon release when the deformity is moderate to severe.

Surgical Procedure

The percutaneous lateral release can be done by means of a lateral paratendinous extensor hallucis longus or a first web space (1WS) portal. The first tends to release the complete lateral capsule and the lateral collateral ligament in order to reach the adductor tendon. The 1WS portal tries to preserve the collateral lateral ligament and to release the adductor tendon. Next, the adductor tendon release is explained.

Percutaneous adductor tendon release technique

Using a no.15 blade, a 1WS portal is made at the level of the first metatarsal articular surface (**Fig. 6**A). The blade is progressed with a frontal orientation from 45° to 60° (depending on lateral collateral ligament section) (**Fig. 6**B) until less than a quarter of the blade is inside the joint (**Fig. 6**C). After this, an external rotation is applied to reach the adductor tendon, which is then sectioned with a frontal movement of the blade, and the first toe is directed into varus until the tendon is released (**Fig. 6**D).

SUMMARY

This article provides a comprehensive overview of the published studies and clearly shows that percutaneous lateral release techniques are useful and effective. Adductor tendon percutaneous release seems to be the most used procedure in order to help osteotomies and correct HV deformities, and the percutaneous approach is the authors' recommended technique when a lateral release is needed.

However, because minimally invasive surgery has an extensive learning curve, specific cadaveric training is mandatory for any surgeon considering performing percutaneous procedures. This training is vital in avoiding complications and shortening the surgeon's learning curve.

DISCLOSURE

The authors have nothing to disclose.

REFERENCES

1. Perera AM, Mason L, Stephens MM. The pathogenesis of hallux valgus. J Bone Joint Surg Am 2011;93(17):1650–61.

2. Lucas Y, Hernandez J, Golanó P, et al. Treatment of moderate hallux valgus by percutaneous, extra-articular reverse-L Chevron (PERC) osteotomy. Bone Joint J 2016;98B(3):365–73.

3. Biz C, Fosser M, Dalmau-Pastor M, et al. Functional and radiographic outcomes of hallux valgus correction by mini-invasive surgery with Reverdin-Isham and Akin percutaneous osteotomies: A longitudinal prospective study with a 48-month follow-up. J Orthop Surg Res 2016;11(1). https://doi.org/10.1186/s13018-016-0491-x.

4. Gicquel T, Fraisse B, Marleix S, et al. Percutaneous hallux valgus surgery in children: Short-term outcomes of 33 cases. Orthop Traumatol Surg Res 2013;99(4): 433–9.
5. Scala A, Vendettuoli D. Modified minimal incision subcapital osteotomy for hallux valgus correction. Foot Ankle Spec 2013;6(1):65–72.
6. Jowett CRJ, Bedi HS. Preliminary results and learning curve of the minimally invasive chevron akin operation for hallux valgus. J Foot Ankle Surg 2017;56(3): 445–52.
7. Crespo Romero E, Peñuela Candel R, Gómez S, et al. Percutaneous forefoot surgery for treatment of hallux valgus deformity: an intermediate prospective study. Musculoskelet Surg 2017;101(2):167–72.
8. Siclari A, Decantis V. Arthroscopic lateral release and percutaneous distal osteotomy for hallux valgus: a preliminary report. Foot Ankle Int 2009;30(7):675–9.
9. Brogan K, Lindisfarne E, Akehurst H, et al. Minimally invasive and open distal chevron osteotomy for mild to moderate hallux valgus. Foot Ankle Int 2016; 37(11):1197–204.
10. Díaz Fernández R. Percutaneous triple and double osteotomies for the treatment of hallux valgus. Foot Ankle Int 2017;38(2):159–66.
11. Martínez-Nova A, Sánchez-Rodríguez R, Gómez-Martín B, et al. The effect of adductor tendon transposition in the modified McBride procedure. Foot Ankle Spec 2008;1(5):275–9.
12. Cervi S, Fioruzzi A, Bisogno L, et al. Percutaneous surgery of allux valgus: risks and limitation in our experience. Acta Biomed 2014;85:107–12.
13. Pichierri P, Sicchiero P, Fioruzzi A, et al. Percutaneous hallux valgus surgery: Strengths and weakness in our clinical experience. Acta Biomed 2014;85:121–5.
14. Bauer T, de Lavigne C, Biau D, et al. Percutaneous Hallux Valgus Surgery: A Prospective Multicenter Study of 189 Cases. Orthop Clin North Am 2009;40(4): 505–14.
15. Bauer T, Biau D, Lortat-Jacob A, et al. Percutaneous hallux valgus correction using the Reverdin-Isham osteotomy. Orthop Traumatol Surg Res 2010;96(4): 407–16.
16. Di Giorgio L, Touloupakis G, Simone S, et al. The Endolog system for moderate-to-severe hallux valgus. J Orthop Surg (Hong Kong) 2013;21(1):47–50.
17. Carvalho P, Viana G, Flora M, et al. Percutaneous hallux valgus treatment: Unilaterally or bilaterally. Foot Ankle Surg 2016;22(4):248–53.
18. Martínez-Nova A, Sánchez-Rodríguez R, Leal-Muro A, et al. Dynamic plantar pressure analysis and midterm outcomes in percutaneous correction for mild hallux valgus. J Orthop Res 2011;29(11):1700–6.
19. Kurashige T, Suzuki S. Effectiveness of percutaneous proximal closing wedge osteotomy with akin osteotomy to correct severe hallux valgus determined by radiographic parameters: a 22-month follow-up. Foot Ankle Spec 2016;10(2):170–9.
20. Ahn JH, Choy WS, Lee KW. Arthroscopy of the first metatarsophalangeal joint in 59 consecutive cases. J Foot Ankle Surg 2012;51(2):161–7.
21. Lee M, Walsh J, Smith MM, et al. Hallux valgus correction comparing percutaneous chevron/akin (PECA) and open scarf/akin osteotomies. Foot Ankle Int 2017;38(8):838–46.
22. De Lavigne C, Rasmont Q, Hoang B. Percutaneous double metatarsal osteotomy for correction of severe hallux valgus deformity. Acta Orthop Belg 2011;77(4): 516–21.
23. Lui TH, Ling SKK, Yuen SCP. Endoscopic-assisted correction of hallux valgus deformity. Sports Med Arthrosc 2016;24(1):e8–13.

24. Lui TH, Chan KB, Chow HT, et al. Arthroscopy-assisted correction of hallux valgus deformity. Arthroscopy 2008;24(8):875–80.

25. Shereff MJ, Bejjani FJ, Kummer FJ. Kinematics of the first metatarsophalangeal joint. J Bone Joint Surg Am 1986;68(3):392–8.

26. Haines RW, McDougall A. The anatomy of hallux valgus. J Bone Joint Surg Br 1954;36(2):272–93.

27. McCormick JJ, Anderson RB. The great toe: failed turf toe, chronic turf toe, and complicated sesamoid injuries. Foot Ankle Clin 2009;14(2):135–50.

28. Alvarez R, Haddad RJ, Gould N, et al. The simple bunion: anatomy at the meta-tarsophalangeal joint of the great toe. Foot Ankle 1984;4(5):229–40.

29. Heubach F. Ueber Hallux valgus und seine operative Behandlung nach Edm. Rose. Deutsche Zeitschrift fü Crhirurgie 1897;46:210.

30. Stokes IA, Hutton WC, Stott JR, et al. Forces under the hallux valgus foot before and after surgery. Clin Orthop Relat Res 1979;142:64–72.

31. Nigg BM. Biomechanical aspects of running. In: Nigg BM, editor. Biomechanics of running shoes. Champaign (IL): Human Kinetics Publishers; 1986. p. 1–25.

32. Biz C, Corradin M, Petretta I, et al. Endolog technique for correction of hallux valgus: A prospective study of 30 patients with 4-year follow-up. J Orthop Surg Res 2015;10(1):1–13.

33. Giannini S, Vannini F, Faldini C, et al. The minimally invasive hallux valgus correc-tion (S.E.R.I.). Interact Surg 2007;2(1):17–23.

34. Tong CK, Ho YF. Use of minimally invasive distal metatarsal osteotomy for correc-tion of hallux valgus. J Orthop Trauma Rehabil 2012;16(1):16–21.

35. Maffulli N, Longo UG, Oliva F, et al. Bosch osteotomy and scarf osteotomy for hallux valgus correction. Orthop Clin North Am 2009;40(4):515–24.

36. Lin YC, Cheng YM, Chang JK, et al. Minimally invasive distal metatarsal osteot-omy for mild-to-moderate hallux valgus deformity. Kaohsiung J Med Sci 2009; 25(8):431–7.

37. Bai LB, Lee KB, Seo CY, et al. Distal Chevron osteotomy with distal soft tissue pro-cedure for moderate to severe hallux valgus deformity. Foot Ankle Int 2010;31: 683–8.

38. Granberry WM, Hickey CH. Hallux valgus correction with metatarsal osteotomy: effect of a lateral distal soft tissue procedure. Foot Ankle Int 1995;16(3):132–8.

39. Yammine K, Assi C. A meta-analysis of comparative clinical studies of isolated osteotomy versus osteotomy with lateral soft tissue release in treating hallux valgus. Foot Ankle Surg 2019;25(5):684–90.

40. Barg A, Harmer JR, Presson AP, et al. Unfavorable outcomes following surgical treatment of hallux valgus deformity: a systematic literature review. J Bone Joint Surg Am 2018;100(18):1563–73.

41. Bock P, Kluger R, Kristen KH. The Scarf osteotomy with minimally invasive lateral release for treatment of hallux valgus deformity: intermediate and long-term re-sults. J Bone Joint Surg Am 2015;97(15):1238–45.

42. de Las Heras-Romero J, Lledó-Alvarez AM, Andrés-Grau J, et al. A new minimally extended distal Chevron osteotomy (MEDCO) with percutaneous soft tissue release (PSTR) for treatment of moderate hallux valgus. Foot (Edinb) 2019;40: 27–33.

43. Maniglio M, Fornaciari P, Bäcker H, et al. Surgical treatment of mild to severe hallux valgus deformities with a percutaneous subcapital osteotomy combined with a lateral soft tissue procedure. Foot Ankle Spec 2019;12(2):138–45.

44. Park YB, Lee KB, Kim SK, et al. Comparison of distal soft-tissue procedures com-bined with a distal chevron osteotomy for moderate to severe hallux valgus: first

web-space versus transarticular approach. J Bone Joint Surg Am 2013;95(21): e158.

45. Grle M, Vrgoc G, Bohacek I, et al. Surgical treatment of moderate hallux valgus: a comparison of distal chevron metatarsal osteotomy with and without lateral soft-tissue release. Foot Ankle Spec 2017;10(6):524–30.

46. Lee HJ, Chung JW, Chu IT, et al. Comparison of distal chevron osteotomy with and without lateral soft tissue release for the treatment of hallux valgus. Foot Ankle Int 2010;31(4):291–5.

47. Kim HN, Suh DH, Hwang PS, et al. Role of intraoperative varus stress test for lateral soft tissue release during chevron bunion procedure. Foot Ankle Int 2011;32(4):362–7.

48. Vernois J, Redfern DJ. Percutaneous surgery for severe hallux valgus. Foot Ankle Clin 2016;21(3):479–93.

49. de Cesar Netto C, Roberts LE, Hudson PW, et al. The success rate of first metatarsophalangeal joint lateral soft tissue release through a medial transarticular approach: A cadaveric study. Foot Ankle Surg 2019;25(6):733–73.

50. Lucattelli G, Catani O, Sergio F, et al. Preliminary experience with a minimally invasive technique for hallux valgus correction with no fixation. Foot Ankle Int 2020;41(1):37–43.

51. Seki H, Suda Y, Takeshima K, et al. Minimally invasive distal linear metatarsal osteotomy combined with selective release of lateral soft tissue for severe hallux valgus. J Orthop Sci 2018;23(3):557–64.

Fixation Principles in Minimal Incision Hallux Valgus Surgery

David B. Kay, MD

KEYWORDS

- Minimal incision surgery • Hallus valgus surgery • Corrective bunion surgery

KEY POINTS

- Greater translation of the distal metatarsal negates the intrinsic stability of chevron and scarf type osteotomies.
- Fixation of the osteotomy becomes more critical and technically difficult with greater translations.
- There are few studies that compare fixation methods with greater than 50% translation.

INTRODUCTION

The purpose of corrective bunion surgery is to relieve the pain associated with the first metatarsal head medial prominence.[1,2] Because of both patient and surgeon dissatisfaction with the results of traditional surgical interventions, there is a revitalized and concerted effort to change the approach to surgical management to improve outcomes.[3] These outcomes concern the pain of the acute procedure, the healing time, the recurrence incidence, the time to full weight-bearing in shoes, the time to return to activities, and stiffness. The surgeon also has other outcomes; these include the reliability and reproducibility of the procedure as well as costs. The costs can be calculated in training time, intraoperative time, materials costs, follow-up care, the recurrence costs, and patient satisfaction costs. There are few published studies on the stability of osteotomies with extensive lateral translation and minimal bone contact.[4,5] There are few published studies on mechanical constructs with extensive lateral translations.[6] This article outlines the constructs associated with distal first metatarsal osteotomies using minimal incision surgical (MIS) techniques.

Orthopedic Surgery, Northeast Ohio Medical University, 3975 Embassy Parkway, Akron, OH 44333, USA
E-mail address: dbkay50@gmail.com

Foot Ankle Clin N Am 25 (2020) 385–398
https://doi.org/10.1016/j.fcl.2020.05.011
1083-7515/20/© 2020 Elsevier Inc. All rights reserved.

foot.theclinics.com

SURGICAL PROCEDURE SELECTION

There are many described surgical techniques for the correction of bunion deformity. It is paramount that the deformity is clearly defined. These factors include the following:

- Foot type, cavus or pes planus
- Mobility of the medial column, with attention to the first tarsometatarsal joint
- Pain at the first tarsometatarsal joint
- Pronation of the metatarsal head
- Mobility of the first metatarsal phalangeal joint
- Pain at the first metatarsal phalangeal joint
- Hallux valgus interphalangeus
- Sesamoid pain
- Thickness of the medial capsule
- Character of the medial eminence that may require excision
- Can the deformity be passively corrected?
- Associated forefoot conditions, including plantar plate instability, windswept toes, neuromuscular imbalance, metatarsus adductus, and extrinsic and intrinsic tendon imbalance
- Posterior compartment contracture

RADIOGRAPHIC CRITERIA

- The width of the first and second intermetatarsal space
- The width of the first metatarsal at the osteotomy site
- Presence of cysts within the metatarsal head
- Bone quality
- Presence of arthritis with staging
- Sesamoid location and presence of sesamoid arthritis
- Pronation of the metatarsal head
- Metatarsus adductus
- Instability of the first metatarsocuneiform joint
- Alignment of the distal metatarsal articular angle, neutral or valgus
- Width and character of the medial eminence

Other physical findings should demonstrate normal vascularity, sensation, and motor function. Medical conditions that interfere with healing would include tobacco use, obesity, and an inability to use gait assistive devices.

SURGICAL APPROACH

Distal osteotomies can be performed with a clear easy-to-visualize open or classic approach. The classic method is to perform a "chevron" or "V"-shaped osteotomy that is centered in the metatarsal head.[7–10] The translation is limited to no more than 50% the width of the metatarsal head. The medial eminence is typically excised, and the capsular repair provides stability. Originally, no internal fixation was used because of the stability of the osteotomy. Over time, this has changed from suture to Kirschner wire(s) or screw(s). The fixation has been placed both dorsal-proximal to plantar-distal or dorsal-distal to plantar-proximal. The osteotomy has been changed from equidistant dorsal and plantar limbs to asymmetric limbs. The longer limbs require more surgical dissection not only to perform the osteotomy but also to allow for translation. Scarf-shaped osteotomies, another intrinsically stable osteotomy, when the limbs are shortened is a distal osteotomy.[11]

The traditional chevron procedure is reliable, reproducible, and stable; however, it is very limited in the correction capabilities.[12–15] If the distal metatarsal articular angle is to be corrected, then additional osteotomies must be performed. It is not possible to rotate the metatarsal head and the limited translation is only effective for mild deformities.[16] Soft tissue balancing is also limited. The intracapsular osteotomy combined with medial and lateral soft tissue imbrication and release, respectively, may result in avascular necrosis or increased stiffness.[17,18] Once these restraints, limited translation, and a reliance on soft tissue release, were challenged, the fixation requirements became more important. An unintended consequence is to have a cosmetically acceptable foot, but one that is stiff, painful, and nonfunctional.

Primary bone healing is a fundamental principle in orthopedic surgery. However, foot and ankle surgery challenges this by open wedge, crescentic, and translational osteotomies that have little native bone contact and/or inherent stability. Therefore, the constructs must provide enough inherent stability without relying on the geometry of the osteotomy. The loading to the bone is significant and complex. Anatomically, the implants are positioned on the dorsum of the foot or the medial column. Plantar positioning is ideal because this is the tension side of the bone during loading; however, the anatomic access is challenging. The mechanical stability is further challenged by the release of the plantar structures that may be necessary for deformity correction.

The placement of the fixation implants should capture the highest quality bone that is usually in the subchondral or periarticular region. The anatomic curves and obliquity can make placement difficult especially when using MIS approaches. Implants placed into joints or even wires placed across joints for temporary fixation will lead to articular damage. Ideally, the implants should not be noticeable to the patient. Replacing a bone prominence with an implant prominence must be avoided.[19–23]

IMPLANT DESIGN AND SELECTION

Surgical implant design must be able to achieve all of the following surgical goals:

- Reliable
- Reproducible
- Ease of use of the implants and instruments
- Standardized implant instrumentation
- Simplification
- Movement to outpatient surgery centers
- Unintended consequences
- Costs
- Learning curve
- Mechanical robustness
- Adaptability
- Removable
- Limited radiation exposure

RELIABLE

Surgical procedures need to be reliable with predictable results. The disability associated with sustainable bunion procedures is significant. The procedure cannot fail during any stage. The preoperative planning should be straightforward with key elements measured. Superfluous information can lead to unneeded interventions.

Intraoperative failure from poor design, fabrication, or execution should not occur. Of course, the surgeon should not modify a procedure that has been carefully designed and tested.

REPRODUCIBLE

Procedures must be reproducible. A procedure should not only be reproducible in a single surgeon's hands but among all surgeons performing the procedure. This is achieved by a reduction in the technique to the essential steps. Every motion and maneuver must be carefully planned to move the procedure to the end goal. Prolonged anesthesia and tourniquet use must be avoided. There must be no waste. Proper planning of deformity will allow for selection of the preferred procedure. The planning needs to take into account the patient expectations. A postoperative radiograph that demonstrates a straight toe is only one parameter. The better question may be how does this foot function, even without complete correction.[11,24-35]

EASE OF USE OF THE IMPLANTS AND INSTRUMENTS

There will be multiple steps in a procedure, limitations in one of the repetitive steps impacts the overall result. For example, let us look at the placement of a cannulated screw. A determination of the implant starting and ending point with trajectory must be calculated. The guidewire is placed. This wire may be in an instrument/implant caddy or may be in a presterilized container. Either way, the wire size and type are determined and then placed into a keyless or keyed chuck. The wire length must not be so short that there is not sufficient length to completely drive the wire or left so long that it is not controllable and wanders on insertion. A cannula may be used. The wire is placed, then the position is verified, typically with fluoroscopy with multiple images. The length is measured, the wire may be driven through the opposite side and then grasped with an instrument so it will not be removed with the drilling. Drilling is followed by countersinking and then screw selection is made with an estimation for countersinking depth and compression. The thread length is also estimated. The screw is placed over the guidewire and then inserted. Once the screw is inserted, another series of fluoroscopic images is taken to verify placement. The guidewire is now removed. The insertion of a cannulated screw involves multiple steps and is a staple of MIS surgery. Simplification has occurred by instruments that measure and countersink the screw. Screws can be self-drilling with varying degrees of success depending on bone quality. The drilling threads typically provide minimal bone capture and if they perforate the opposite side of the bone, the sharp edges can damage the soft tissues. Screws have many driver configurations, including square, hex, cruciform, or torx type. The lack of standardization can make for a high level of complexity on removal. Screwdriver handles also influence ease of use. A handle that is too small is difficult to hold and one that is too large can generate much torque that may be inappropriate. A large handle may be difficult to hold for a small hand, and if the screwdriver shaft is long, then the surgeon is isolated from the "feel" of the screw as it is being driven into the bone. A simple handle is constantly regripped with a momentary loss of the driver engagement and a potential to strip the screw head. The constant regripping can lead to wobble on screw insertion that will increase heat generation and tear the bone. These factors can lead to local inflammation that may cause screw loosening with a premature loss of fixation. These are all basic repetitive tasks that are complicated by MIS when visualization cues are absent.

STANDARDIZED IMPLANT INSTRUMENTATION

Orthopedic screws were initially introduced with very simple recessed slots and "X" shapes for the screwdriver interface. These subsequently gave way to hex-shaped recesses that were the standard for many years. Torx-shaped recesses have become common and provide an excellent interface; however, we now have a variety of other implant driver shapes that are proprietary. Small and micro screws are difficult to handle, whether they are opened one at a time from a container or removed from a tray. The lack of standards in screw recesses is problematic for the surgeon and the surgical staff.

SIMPLIFICATION

Simplification, doing only what is necessary to reach the goal, is essential for reliability and reproducibility of a surgical procedure.[22] The starting point in simplification is a clear understanding of the problem. The "problem" may be pain to the medial eminence, pain in the joint, numbness of the toe, irritation of the second toe, crossover second toe, unstable metatarsocuneiform (MTC) joint also associated with an incompetent medial column, or an arthritic MTC or metatarsophalangeal joint. There may be combinations of the described "problems" that all need to be addressed.[36,37] The "problem" for many is just a foot that has a width that makes shoe-wear difficult. Once all of the issues that need to be addressed are identified, then the proper choice of interventions can be chosen. Simplification is doing all that is needed and not more. The concept that MIS is "simple" greatly underestimates the technical skill needed to reliably perform the procedure. Appreciation of the 3-dimensional positioning is critical for alignment of the metatarsal head in proper translation, angulation, and rotation.[38,39] Translations of greater than 50% do not allow for the guardrails and inherent stability of lesser translation. The chevron or scarf-type osteotomy only allows for one plane correction. Our appreciation of the deformities of a "bunion" have been greatly enhanced with 3-dimensional modeling based on computed tomography scans.[32,40–44] We can identify the bony deformities, and locate cystic and degenerative changes. Once the extent of the deformity is identified, bone correction becomes more straightforward; however there are other aspects of the deformity that also must be accounted for: pain location, eminence versus joint pain. First, MTC pain and instability must be assessed. Associated deformities to the lesser toes, midfoot, hindfoot, and ankle. One of the more difficult components to objectively measure is intrinsic and extrinsic muscle strength. The maintenance of the correction is predicated on proper rebalancing of the muscles and tendons. There is little question that extreme muscle imbalance as seen in cerebral palsy is best treated with arthrodesis; however, there may be more subtle motor imbalance that leads to recurrent deformity.

MOVEMENT TO OUTPATIENT SURGERY CENTERS

The location of most surgical procedures has been shifted to outpatient centers. This brings many challenges. The resources of the outpatient centers may be limited by equipment, personnel, and reimbursement. Large containers, consisting of every conceivable implant and instrument are very difficult to sterilize. This becomes a significant problem when the equipment is needed multiple times in 1 day. Reimbursement for the procedure may not cover implant charges. This automatically preselects the most inexpensive implant or completely eliminates the use of any implant. and now relies on external bandages and patient cooperation.

COSTS

A discussion of costs of care is one of the most contentious issues in current medical treatment, regardless of country. Orthopedic care is directed at the implant costs primarily and the surgical fee secondarily; however, other costs seem to be given little attention. These would include time in the operating room, anesthesia costs, and loss of time at work for the patient. Operating room costs are significant and can be attributed to a full staff, including a circulating nurse, surgical technician assistant, and anesthesia and fluoroscopy technician. Reducing the personnel may reduce the direct costs but there may be indirect cost increases, particularly inefficacies and poor time utilization. The physical environment is one of the design inputs that must be taken into account.

UNINTENDED CONSEQUENCES

Unintended consequences are just a fact of life. All of the planning, care, and attention to detail on the part of the design team will be negated when unintended consequences occur. Some are preventable and can actually be anticipated and some cannot. Surgeons have a habit of modifying procedures that they have never performed and toss their training time. Hospitals will substitute materials for a cost savings and the components will not properly fit together. A generic drill bit may be used that is undersized or oversized for the screws. Patients are notorious for not following postoperative instructions. It is critical for post market surveillance to better understand the results that occur and to adapt to the unintended or unanticipated consequences.

LEARNING CURVE

The dreaded learning curve is important in the adoption and proper application of the procedure. This starts with a clear understanding of the problem and how the procedure is optimally applied. This would be the didactic component of the training. It is important that the information is concise, clearly presented, and unbiased. All too often a new procedure is presented as the only solution when, in fact, it is only intended to address a specific problem. Too much information only confuses the users and too little does not allow for proper utilization. When the complexity of the procedure is not improved through the integrated instrumentation and implant design, only a limited adoption occurs.[45] If the physical training is not augmented through additional readily available refresher training tools, additional burdens are created. The learning curve creates uncertainty for the surgeon and results that will not match the results from the design team. Learning and adopting a new procedure initially involves a leap of faith. MIS is further complicated by the lack of visual, tactile, and even auditory feedback.

MECHANICAL ROBUSTNESS

Most of the attention, at the introduction of a new implant system, is the touting of a mechanically robust system. Testing that has been carefully designed shows how much "stronger" the new system is over current systems. This is a very flawed method for introduction and is only relevant when the current choices are both mechanically and clinically inferior. The stated goal of many systems is to allow for immediate weight-bearing. Immediate weight-bearing is very attractive to prevent what has been termed "fracture disease." Fracture disease results in muscle and skin atrophy, reduced endurance, and disuse osteoporosis. However, we are creating osteotomies that have little intrinsic stability, and in an individual who is high risk for nonunion, the weight-bearing process must be properly modified. Those who use tobacco, are obese, steroid dependent, osteoporotic, or do not have the ability to follow instructions will benefit from a delay in weight-bearing. We also have to be wary of stress shielding that occurs when the bone is not loaded as a source of nonunion. When performing a greater than 50% up to a 100% lateral translation of a distal osteotomy, care must be taken to assess for cystic changes in the metatarsal head. Even a large screw will not have significant purchase with a cyst. The screws used in a percutaneous chevron akin or minimally invasive chevron akin (MICA/PECA) procedure should not compress the capital fragment. Compression will change the alignment and there may be so little direct bone contact that this should be avoided. There is very little published on the tipping point where bone surface contact is no longer relevant. The traditional method of stabilization in a limited chevron, is to place 1 or 2 screws oriented from dorsal to plantar. When there is minimal translation and significant bone surface contact, the screw placement is straightforward. Kirschner wires are effective when there is more than 50% contact surface. When the translation is 50% or greater, the "window" for implant positioning is challenging, as illustrated in **Fig. 1**. The overhanging bone is typically excised to further complicate the placement of traditional screws. MICA/PECA screw placement is directed from proximal medial to distal lateral. Typically, 2 screws are placed for rotational control. Accurate and consistent placement of the screws can be challenging even for skilled surgeons.[4,5,46,47] Another approach is to build an intramedullary support and attach screws to the capital fragment. Different methods have been described for both the extended distal osteotomy and a scarf osteotomy that leverages the intramedullary canal as a support structure.[48–51] The intramedullary placement allows for limited incisions to insert devices that may be equivalent to plating. The intramedullary placement will not cause soft tissue irritation that occurs with standard plates and even screw heads. These devices would include the ISO, Endolog, Stofella, and the V-Tek. **Table 1** provides a broad overview of the implant selection that is available at the time this article was prepared. **Fig. 1** demonstrates the contact surface of the bone after translation. The greater the shift, the less the contact and the greater the obliquity of the screws. **Fig. 2** demonstrates a significant translation stabilized by an intramedullary/extra-osseous implant. The transverse screws are locking to provide fixation when the cysts in the metatarsal head reduce the bone quality.

ADAPTABILITY

Anatomic variability is a given and the implants must be adaptable for each individual. Screws must be able to purchase bone that is dense and osteoporotic. Screw heads must be designed not to irritate tendons and skin. Plates must be able to be contoured and still be stable. It is unlikely that there will be a "perfect" fit out of the case. Although screws and Kirschner wires are very adaptable, this creates variability in the placement of the implants. Jigs have been created for osteotomy placement as well as fixation alignment. Jig placement can be challenging with small bones of the foot and obtaining proper 3-dimensional alignment.

REMOVABLE

Implants need to be removable under a variety of circumstances that include nonunion, improper placement, infection, soft tissue irritation, patient preference for removal, reaction to the implant, and conversion to another procedure. An example would be a distal first metatarsal osteotomy that results in avascular necrosis or osteoarthritis. Conversion to an arthrodesis should not be further complicated

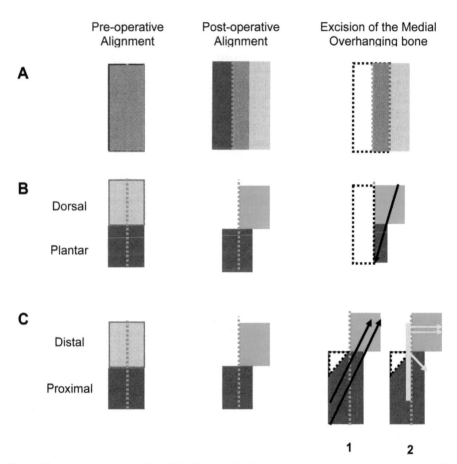

Fig. 1. The bone contact surface. (*A*) View of the bone from a typical anteroposterior (AP) radiograph. The green dotted line is the midline. The black dotted line is the overhanging bone that is removed. (*B*) Perspective of a chevron-type distal metatarsal osteotomy. The arrow is the screw orientation from dorsal to plantar and represents the very small plantar bone remaining. This is a 50% lateral translation. (*C*) 1 is an MICA screw placement as viewed on an AP radiograph and demonstrates the minimal bone contact and screw orientation with a 50% lateral translation. 2 is the same model with an intra/extramedullary implant.

by the inability to remove the implants or have a defect that may require staged procedures or custom implants. The lack of standard screw recesses presents another challenge of having the correct tools. Locking screws that are "cold welded" into the plate must also be avoided. Driver recesses must be designed for removal as well as insertion.

RADIATION EXPOSURE

Radiation exposure must be minimized to the surgeon, patient, and operating room staff. MIS requires fluoroscopic imaging to visualize the instrument insertion and alignment, positioning of the osteotomized bone fragments, and temporary and permanent fixation placement must be verified. It is common that the surgeon's hands will receive

Table 1 Generic implants			
Type of Fixation	**Advantages**	**Disadvantages**	**MIS Applicable**
Suture/Stainless steel wire	Inexpensive, readily available	Poor mechanical stability	Limited
Kirschner wire - capture	Inexpensive, readily available and adaptable	May not provide adequate stabilization. Percutaneous placement can cause skin irritation.	Can be used, but the stiffness/diameter must be matched to the needed stability.
Kirschner wire – Abutment	Inexpensive, readily available and adaptable	Relies on abutment of the wire to maintain the translation. No rotational control. No translational control	Clinical studies showing application
Cannulated screw; headed	Relatively inexpensive. Easy to use. Must balance guide wire stiffness to screw wall diameter.	Head must be countersunk.	Commonly used
Cannulated screw; headless	Relatively inexpensive. Easy to use. Must balance guide wire stiffness to screw wall diameter.	Head may need to be countersunk. Bone overgrowth of the head can make removal difficult.	Commonly used
Plate and screws	Readily available in generic form	Limited application because of the exposure needed for implantation.	Limited use
Staple	Static staples are inexpensive and readily available. Compression staples can cause displacement with extreme capital shifts	Exposure is needed for insertion and is limited for MIS.	Limited use

Abbreviation: MIS, minimal incision surgery.

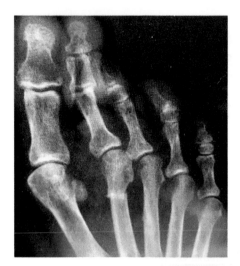
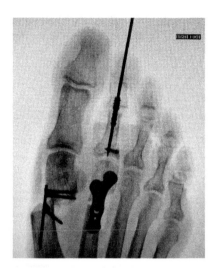

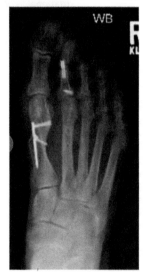

Fig. 2. Preoperative image of a recurrent hallux valgus with a 100% translation stabilized with an intramedullary plate system. Immediate postsurgical and 1-year follow-up.

radiation exposure. Proper planning, simplicity, experience, and execution will be critical in reducing the exposure.

FUTURE

The future of bunion correction would include patient-specific guides or navigation. The preoperative planning will allow for a variety of determinations that would include the following:

- A 3-dimensional model of the foot that can be used to simulate the procedure and create a patient-specific plan and guides.

- A precise evaluation of the rotation, sagittal, and coronal components to determine the final position of the metatarsal head.
- Determination of preoperative sesamoid placement that evaluates sesamoid morphology once reduced.
- Evaluation of the neuromuscular function of the intrinsic and extrinsic musculature.
- Understanding specific bone healing capacity with modulation if needed.
- Implants that incorporate into the bone.
- Restoration of joints to limit fusion procedures.

SUMMARY
Purpose of These Categories

Implant design is an increasingly complex task that follows a simple directive, "Do more, do better with less." These categories are only some of the design inputs that must be addressed in our resource-constrained environment. All too often, there is a single input that is used for implant design. All of the members of the care team must be aligned to achieve these goals. We are in a period of reevaluation of the results of this common surgery and only time will allow us to objectively evaluate the results. Some of the procedures will be abandoned, some modified, and some widely adopted. We must all be objective and honest in our appraisals of the procedures and not follow the mistakes of the past.

DISCLOSURE

The author is a consultant to Wright Medical.

REFERENCES

1. Perera AM, Mason L, Stephens MM. The pathogenesis of hallux valgus. J Bone Joint Surg Am 2011;93(17):1650–61.
2. Piggott H. The natural history of hallux valgus in adolescence and early adult life. J Bone Joint Surg Br 1960;42(4):749.
3. Barg A, Harmer JR, Presson AP, et al. Unfavorable outcomes following surgical treatment of hallux valgus deformity: a systematic literature review. J Bone Joint Surg Am 2018;100(18):1563–73.
4. Buciuto R. Prospective randomized study of chevron osteotomy versus Mitchell's osteotomy in hallux valgus. Foot Ankle Int 2014;35(12):1268–76.
5. Chiang CC, Lin CFJ, Tzeng YH, et al. Distal linear osteotomy compared to oblique diaphyseal osteotomy in moderate to severe hallux valgus. Foot Ankle Int 2012; 33(6):479–86.
6. Kugan R, Currall VA, Johal P, et al. The foot proximal first metatarsal opening wedge osteotomy: geometric analysis on saw bone models. Foot (Edinb) 2015; 25(1):1–4.
7. Trnka HJ. Osteotomies for hallux valgus correction. Foot Ankle Clin N Am 2005; 10:15–33.
8. Trnka HJ, Zembsch A, Easley ME, et al. The chevron osteotomy for correction of hallux valgus. Comparison of findings after two and five years of follow-up. J Bone Joint Surg Am 2000;82-A(10):1373–8.
9. Donnelly R, Saltzman C, Todd K, et al. Modified chevron osteotomy for hallux valgus. Foot Ankle Int 1994;15:642–5.

10. Austin DW, Leventen EO. A new osteotomy for hallux valgus: a horizontally directed "v" displacement osteotomy of the metatarsal head for hallux valgus and primus varus. Clin Orthop Relat Res 1981;157:25–30.

11. Lai MC, Rikhraj IS, Woo YL, et al. Clinical and radiological outcomes comparing percutaneous chevron-akin osteotomies vs open scarf-akin osteotomies for hallux valgus. Foot Ankle Int 2018;39(3):311–7.

12. McCarthy AD, Davies MB, Wembridge KR, et al. Three-dimensional analysis of different first metatarsal osteotomies in a hallux valgus model. Foot Ankle Int 2008;29(6):606–12.

13. Prado M, Baumfeld T, Nery C, et al. Rotational biplanar chevron osteotomy. Foot Ankle Surg 2019. https://doi.org/10.1016/j.fas.2019.05.011.

14. Radwan YA, Mansour AMR. Percutaneous distal metatarsal osteotomy versus distal chevron osteotomy for correction of mild-to-moderate hallux valgus deformity. Arch Orthop Trauma Surg 2012;132(11):1539–46.

15. Seki H, Suda Y, Takeshima K, et al. Minimally invasive distal linear metatarsal osteotomy combined with selective release of lateral soft tissue for severe hallux valgus. J Orthop Sci 2018;23(3):557–64.

16. Saltzman CL, Brandser EA, Anderson CM, et al. Coronal plane rotation of the first metatarsal. Foot Ankle Int 1996;17(3):157–61.

17. Edwards WH. Avascular necrosis of the first metatarsal head. Foot Ankle Clin Rev 2005;10(1):117–27.

18. Park YB, Lee KB, Kim SK, et al. Comparison of distal soft-tissue procedures combined with a distal chevron osteotomy for moderate to severe hallux valgus: first web-space versus transarticular approach. J Bone Joint Surg Am 2013;95(21):e158.

19. Giannini S, Faldini C, Nanni M, et al. A minimally invasive technique for surgical treatment of hallux valgus: simple, effective, rapid, inexpensive (SERI). Int Orthop 2013;37(9):1805–13.

20. Wagner E, Ortiz C. Osteotomy considerations in hallux valgus treatment: improving the correction power. Foot Ankle Clin 2012;17(3):481–98.

21. Di Giorgio L, Touloupakis G, Simone S, et al. The Endolog system for moderate-to-severe hallux valgus. J Orthop Surg (Hong Kong) 2013;21(1):47–50.

22. Bösch P, Wanke S, Legenstein R. Hallux valgus correction by the method of Bösch: a new technique with a seven-to-ten-year follow-up. Foot Ankle Clin 2000;5(3):485–98.

23. Giannini S, Ceccarelli F, Bevoni R, et al. Hallux valgus surgery: the minimally invasive bunion correction (SERI). Tech Foot Ankle Surg 2003;2:11–20.

24. Okuda R, Kinoshita M. Postoperative incomplete reduction of the sesamoids as a risk factor for recurrence of hallux valgus. J Bone Joint Surg Am 2009;91:1637–45.

25. Heerspink FOL, Verburg H, Reininga IHF, et al. Chevron versus Mitchell osteotomy in hallux valgus surgery: a comparative study. J Foot Ankle Surg 2015;54(3):361–4.

26. Huang PJ, Lin YC, Fu YC, et al. Radiographic evaluation of minimally invasive distal metatarsal osteotomy for hallux valgus. Foot Ankle Int 2011;32(5):503–7.

27. Ianno B, Familiari F, De Gori M, et al. Midterm results and complications after minimally invasive distal metatarsal osteotomy for treatment of hallux valgus. Foot Ankle Int 2013;34(7):969–77.

28. Maffulli N, Longo UG, Marinozzi A, et al. Hallux valgus: effectiveness and safety of minimally invasive surgery. A systematic review. Br Med Bull 2011;97(1):149–67.

29. Maffulli N, Longo UG, Oliva F, et al. Bosch osteotomy and scarf osteotomy for hallux valgus correction. Orthop Clin North Am 2009;40(4):515–24.
30. Magnan B, Bortolazzi R, Samaila E, et al. Percutaneous distal metatarsal osteotomy for correction of hallux valgus. J Bone Joint Surg Am 2006;88(suppl 1): 135–48.
31. Poggio D, Melo R, Botello J, et al. Comparison of postoperative costs of two surgical techniques for hallux valgus (Kramer vs. scarf). Foot Ankle Surg 2015;21(1): 37–41.
32. Su Kim J, Kim Y, Won Young K, et al. A new measure of tibial sesamoid position in hallux valgus in relation to the coronal rotation of the first metatarsal in CT scans. Foot Ankle Int 2015;36(8):944–52.
33. Yamaguchi S, Sasho T, Endo J, et al. Shape of the lateral edge of the first metatarsal head changes depending on the rotation and inclination of the first metatarsal: a study using digitally reconstructed radiographs. J Orthop Sci 2015; 20(5):868–74.
34. Kaipel M, Reissig L, Albrecht L, et al. Risk of damaging anatomical structures during minimally invasive hallux valgus correction (Bösch technique): an anatomical study. Foot Ankle Int 2018;39(11):1355–9.
35. Oh IS, Choi SW, Kim MK, et al. Clinical and radiological results after modified distal metatarsal osteotomy for hallux valgus. Foot Ankle Int 2008;29(5):473–7.
36. Dayton P, Feilmeier M, Kauwe M, et al. Relationship of frontal plane rotation of first metatarsal to proximal articular set angle and hallux alignment in patients undergoing tarsometatarsal arthrodesis for hallux abducto valgus: a case series and critical review of the literature. J Foot Ankle Surg 2013;52(3):348–54.
37. Mavcic B. Geometric analysis of indications for minimally invasive distal metatarsal osteotomy in treatment of hallux valgus. J Orthop Surg Res 2015;10(1):1–7.
38. Schneider W, Knahr K. Metatarsophalangeal and intermetatarsal angle: different values and interpretation of postoperative results dependent on the technique of measurement. Foot Ankle Int 1998;19(8):532–6.
39. Beischer AD, Anat D, Ammon P, et al. Three-dimensional computer analysis of the modified Ludloff osteotomy. Foot Ankle Int 2005;26(8):627–32.
40. Collan L, Kankare JA, Mattila K. The biomechanics of the first metatarsal bone in hallux valgus: a preliminary study utilizing a weight bearing extremity CT. Foot Ankle Surg 2013;19(3):155–61.
41. Cruz EP, Wagner FV, Henning C, et al. Comparison between simple radiographic and computed tomographic three-dimensional reconstruction for evaluation of the distal metatarsal articular angle. J Foot Ankle Surg 2017;56(3):505–9.
42. Kimura T, Kubota M, Taguchi T, et al. Evaluation of first-ray mobility in patients with hallux valgus using weight-bearing CT and a 3-D analysis system. J Bone Joint Surg Am 2017;99:247–55.
43. Ota T, Nagura T, Kokubo T, et al. Etiological factors in hallux valgus, a three-dimensional analysis of the first metatarsal. J Foot Ankle Res 2017;10(1):1–6.
44. Seki H, Oki S, Suda Y, et al. Three-dimensional analysis of the first metatarsal bone in minimally invasive distal linear metatarsal osteotomy for hallux valgus. Foot Ankle Int 2019;9:1–10.
45. Giannini S, Cavallo M, Faldini C, et al. The SERI distal metatarsal osteotomy and scarf osteotomy pro- vide similar correction of hallux valgus. Clin Orthop Relat Res 2013;(471):2305–11.
46. Kadakia AR, Smerek JP, Myerson MS. Radiographic results after percutaneous distal metatarsal osteotomy for correction of hallux valgus deformity. Foot Ankle Int 2007;28:355–60.

47. Angthong C, Yoshimura I, Kanazawa K, et al. Minimally invasive distal linear metatarsal osteotomy for correction of hallux valgus: a preliminary study of clinical outcome and analytical radiographic results via a mapping system. Arch Orthop Trauma Surg 2013;133(3):321–31.

48. Biz C, Corradin M, Petretta I, et al. Endolog technique for correction of hallux valgus: a prospective study of 30 patients with 4-year follow-up. J Orthop Surg Res 2015;10:102.

49. Bohnert L, Radeideh A, Bigolin G, et al. Mechanical testing of maximal shift scarf osteotomy with inside-out plating compared to classic scarf osteotomy with double screw fixation. Foot Ankle Surg 2018;57(6):1056–8.

50. Bennett GL, Sabetta JA. Evaluation of an innovative fixation system for chevron bunionectomy. Foot Ankle Int 2016;37(2):205–9.

51. Bennett GL, Klaus D, Shemory S, et al. Intraosseous sliding plate fixation used in double osteotomy bunionectomy. Foot Ankle Int 2019;40(1):85–8.

Complications of Minimally Invasive Surgery for Hallux Valgus and How to Deal with Them

Georg Hochheuser, MD[a,b,c,]*

KEYWORDS

- Hallux valgus • Percutaneous • Minimally invasive • Complications

KEY POINTS

- This article provides a comprehensive overview of the possible complications in minimally invasive surgery (MIS) for hallux valgus.
- In general, the possible complications are the same in MIS as for open surgery and, according to recent data, the rate of complications and the outcomes are at least comparable with open techniques.
- Because of the minor soft tissue trauma and the possibility of immediate full weight bearing, a percutaneous technique provides the best conditions for undisturbed healing.
- In contrast, some specific possible complications can be found in MIS that do not exist in open surgery, such as lesion of soft tissue structures that are not under direct visible control or skin burns.
- These complications are usually the result of technical mistakes in performing the operation. To avoid complications, it is therefore crucial to get proper education in MIS by cadaver training and visiting experienced colleagues, just as is done in open surgery.

INTRODUCTION

Complications following hallux valgus reconstruction have an expected incidence of between 10% to 55%.[1] Complications include undercorrection, overcorrection, recurrence, transfer metatarsalgia, nonunion, malunion, avascular necrosis (AVN), arthritis, hardware removal, nerve injury, and ultimately patient dissatisfaction.[2] A systematic literature review recently showed an overall rate of recurrent deformity of 4.9%,

[a] Chirurgisch Orthopädisches Centrum am diako, Frölichstraße 13, Augsburg 86150, Germany;
[b] GRECMIP soon MIFAS: Minimally Invasive Foot and Ankle Society, 2 Rue Negrevergne, Merignac 33700, France; [c] GFFC: German Society of Foot and Ankle Surgery, Gewerbegebiet 18, Raisting 82399, Germany
* Chirurgisch Orthopädisches Centrum am diako, Frölichstr.13, Augsburg 86391, Germany.
E-mail address: hochheuser@cocd-augsburg.de

Foot Ankle Clin N Am 25 (2020) 399–406
https://doi.org/10.1016/j.fcl.2020.04.002
1083-7515/20/© 2020 Elsevier Inc. All rights reserved.

metatarsalgia of 6.3%, and dissatisfaction of 10.6% from 229 studies published between 1968 and 2016 including various types of open procedures.[3] The rate of revision surgery in open hallux valgus correction varies from 5.5% to 8.8%.[4]

However, in the last few years, more and more minimally invasive procedures were developed for correction of hallux valgus. In Germany, minimally invasive surgery (MIS) is now used by a minority of 7% of foot and ankle surgeons. This rate was shown in a nationwide survey of 427 foot and ankle surgeons.[5] In the meantime, there were more and more articles that showed good results for minimally invasive operations.

The minimally invasive Chevron and Akin (MICA) proved to be a safe and powerful procedure to effectively treat even severe deformities. However, cadaver training is recommended.[6] In a 2-year follow-up study it was shown to be a safe and reliable procedure.[7]

Another study showed results comparable with the open procedure for minimally invasive Chevron osteotomy.[8] Furthermore, the MIS miniscarf is as effective as the standard approach for mild and moderate hallux valgus.[9,10]

Because there is no direct view on the anatomic structures at risk, there was some concern of a higher risk of complications in MIS compared with open surgery. In cadaver studies, it there is only minimal risk of neurovascular and tendon injury associated with minimally invasive techniques in the forefoot.[11] In calcaneal osteotomies, the Shannon burrs have proved to spare the neurovascular structures.[12] In addition to these MIS-specific complications, all the same complications of hallux valgus surgery performed with an open technique can also be observed.

GENERAL COMPLICATIONS
Infection

MIS in general provides the best conditions for uncomplicated wound healing. The small incisions minimize the portals for bacterial infection and preserve local blood supply. In addition, the tourniquet is nonessential and, in experienced hands, a shorter operating-room time can be achieved; these are known positive predictive factors concerning infections.

Hence, the rate of infections in MIS is very low, at 0% to 0.8%.[13,14] In recent publications, the risk of infection is described to be significantly lower than in open surgery.[15] In order to avoid infections, surgeons have to prevent skin burns. If skin burns occur, they are usually caused by technical mistakes such excessive burr speed and/or deficient cooling of the skin by water. The anatomy and resulting incision points have to be identified meticulously. Heating the skin with the running burr must be avoided. The pivoting point of the drill has to be maintained exactly at the skin level to prevent distorting of the skin with translation of the running burr.

In addition, during burr use, constant rinsing with water to cool the skin is required. If skin burns occur, they should be excised at the end of the operation. If infections nevertheless occur, antiinflammatory drugs or antibiotics are usually sufficient for treatment. Surgical procedures in most cases are not necessary.[16]

Moreover, it is important to thoroughly wash out all debris from the surgical site. If small bony particles stay in the wound, they can cause persistent secretions. In these cases, the small splinters have to be removed and the wound will become dry.

If severe infections should occur, they are treated with the same principles as for open surgery.

AVASCULAR NECROSIS

In an anatomic study of surgeons inexperienced in MIS, the risk of iatrogenic injury while performing MIS techniques was assessed. There was no apparent damage to the arterial plexus in any specimen.[11] Another study in 1000 cases of MIS hallux valgus correction showed not a single occurrence of AVN.[17]

However, AVN may be found in lesser metatarsals, where it is a rare complication of distal metatarsal osteotomy just as in open techniques.

The dorsal and plantar arteries form a vascular ring around the heads of lower metatarsals. There is an extensive extraosseous arterial network around the heads. The nutrient arteries enter the heads at the metaphysis near the capsular attachments. In order to avoid AVN, surgeons must know and respect these anatomic findings and stay extra-articular with the osteotomy. This requirement means that, especially with little experience in MIS, the osteotomy should be controlled under fluoroscopy.

If AVN occurs, the strategy of treatment is the same as it would be in open surgery. First nonoperative treatment should be tried, with insoles and so forth. Otherwise the operation has to be redone, usually with open procedures in terms of a closing wedge decompressive osteotomy or with interposition of bony material and osteosynthesis. The final option is that the head could be resected.

DELAYED UNION/NONUNION

Delayed union may be found in the first ray in complete osteotomies with no fixation. In order to prevent it, thermal damage of the bone has to be avoided. Therefore, the surgeon has to take several steps: always work with high torque and low speed (not >6000 rpm) and use new, sharp burrs.

The absence of a tourniquet confers benefit from the cooling effect of the blood. In addition, constant rinsing of water while using the burrs is necessary.

As in MIS, many osteotomies are not fixed, therefore the postoperative dressing becomes very important and has to be done consistently by the surgeon or by specially trained nurses.

Usually delayed union is a purely radiological finding in asymptomatic patients. It has to be noted that, in MIS, the radiological signs of bony healing tend to occur much later than may be expected from open surgery. Surgeons have to be aware of these differences and, also very important, have to explain them to the radiologists they are working with. Otherwise, the radiologist would misinterpret the findings as definite nonunion and may make the patient insecure. If radiologically delayed union occurs, patient and radiologist have to be informed about these findings and their meaning in percutaneous surgery. Vitamin D und calcium can be given, also shock wave therapy can be taken into consideration.

Because most patients are pain free, immobilization usually is not necessary and simple patience is needed. Never act hastily to do a revision because most delayed unions fuse by 12 to 18 months and nonunion occurs only in 0.1 to 0.2%.[18]

NERVE INJURIES

Postoperative dysesthesia is seen frequently in MIS hallux valgus surgery. In the literature, it is described in up to 12% of cases, but, in most cases, this is only a transient phenomenon caused by swelling or bruising of soft tissue.[16] Persistent paresthesia is observed in only 0.5% of cases.[13] In order to avoid lesions of the nerves, detailed anatomic knowledge again is of great use. Recently, there was a so-called clock method introduced, which defined a safe-zone medially and laterally to the extensor hallucis longus tendon.[19]

STIFFNESS

Stiffness of the first metatarsophalangeal (MTP) joint is a common phenomenon after hallux valgus surgery. In open procedures, it is described in between 7% and 38%. A large review of literature on MIS found stiffness of the first MTP overall in 9.8% of cases. Eighteen studies were included, with a total of 1534 procedures for percutaneous hallux valgus surgery.[20]

A recent study compared open scarf and Akin procedures with MIS chevron and Akin and found moderate stiffness in around 6% of cases in both groups.[21]

It could be assumed that, in procedures such as Isham-Reverdin with removal of exostosis and opening of the capsule, the rate of stiffness could be higher than in those procedures that stay extracapsular, such as MIS chevron. However, a recent study in MIS Isham-Reverdin found the rate of postoperative stiffness to be comparable with other percutaneous and open procedures.[22]

However, while performing procedures with opening of the capsule, it is important to concentrate on meticulous removal of all bony debris off the joint. Besides the initial use of rasps, scrupulous washing out of the debris has to be performed. This washing out is best done in an inside-out-technique; that is, a lateral to medial approach. The great toe has to be moved during this maneuver and the washout is continued until the jetting liquid appears crystal clear in order not to leave any debris within the joint. One or, at the latest, 2 weeks after the operation the patients should to instructed to active and passive mobilization of the MTP joint to preserve mobility. Physiotherapy is usually not necessary, and any stiffness usually resolves after physiotherapy.[23]

TENDONS

Tendon injury is extremely rare in MIS. Usually a so-called safe-hole technique is used: the burr is directly introduced into the bone and the cortices are cut from inside the bone (the safe hole). The drill has a characteristic sound as long as it is within bone and a bony structure is being cut. As soon as the burr leaves the bone and reaches soft tissue, that characteristic sound changes. Being attentive to this sensation, the surgeon has a kind of acoustic control of whether the burr is still in the safe hole or not.

In addition, soft tissue structures such as tendons should not be under tension and should not be pressed against the running burr.

The straight burr usually used in hallux valgus surgery does not harm the tendons. However, the conical wedge used, for example, in minimally invasive cheilectomy is more likely to cause injury to tendons, in this case to the extensor hallucis longus. Therefore, it is especially important during this procedure to avoid pressing the tendon against the running burr. In addition, the tendon should be kept relaxed by holding the big toe in dorsiflexion. Some surgeons experienced in MIS lift the tendon to create a working space between tendon and bone and to be sure there is no danger of violating the tendon.

When respecting these principles, lesions of tendons are rare exceptions. If they still occur, they have to be treated the same way as for open surgery.

VASCULAR COMPLICATIONS

Cadaveric studies have shown no damage to the arterial plexus supplying the first metatarsal head, even in inexperienced surgeons.[11] Therefore, arterial bleeding is rarely seen and does not require specific bleeding control. However, if there is an injury to an artery, the blood supply will be secured by the collateral netting.

Because tourniquets are not used, venous bleeding occurs frequently during the operation. If the patient has no problem in blood clotting, no surgical action is required. The bleeding will stop after a short time, and usually even compression is not necessary.

BONY COMPLICATIONS

In MIS, the same complications can be seen as for open surgery. The complications include:

- Undercorrection/recurrence
- Overcorrection
- Transfer metatarsalgia
- Nonunion/malunion
- AVN
- Secondary dislocation

Undercorrection/Recurrence

As for open surgery, there are several different MIS procedures to correct hallux valgus. A gold standard does not exist. The procedure that will achieve good results and avoid recurrence depends on the extent of deformity and the surgeon's experience.

In general, with most surgeons, the Reverdin-Isham procedure covers mild to moderate deformities[22,24] up to an intermetatarsal angle (IMA) of 15° and a hallux valgus angle of 30°. The Reverdin-Isham is always combined with an Akin procedure, and both can be left unfixed. However, some specialists, such as Mariano de Prado,[16] address even much bigger deformities with the Reverdin-Isham and report very good results.

Deformities with an IMA between 15° and 20° can be addressed with a percutaneous chevron osteotomy or double osteotomy; that is, a Reverdin-Isham combined with a basal lateral closing wedge osteotomy, again usually with an additional Akin procedure. For even bigger deformities, MICA has shown good results.

Independently from the procedure chosen, to avoid recurrence it is crucial to correct the proximal articular set angle properly and to have the forces of tendons centered in the joint again. Therefore, in most cases, an additional Akin procedure is recommended. The other main issue in preventing recurrence is careful decision making in terms of which osteotomy to choose for correction of the first metatarsal. If this decision is made correctly and the operation is performed properly, the results will be equal to those of open procedures.[6–10] There is no higher rate of recurrence described in MIS. If there is a symptomatic recurrence, the treatment will have to be a revision just like after open surgery, either in MIS or in an open technique. The procedures chosen again depend on the precise problem and the surgeon's experience.

Secondary Displacement

Secondary displacement can be a specific problem of MIS compared with open surgery, because many MIS osteotomies remain unfixed, which causes no problems as long as the osteotomies are truly closing wedge with 1 cortex untouched and thus stable. However, osteotomies are sometimes complete. These osteotomies occur either accidently, when the surgeon did not manage to spare the second cortex. In other cases, the cutting of the second cortex is intended; for example, to correct an additional rotational malposition of the big toe with a complete Akin osteotomy.

In MIS, it is intended to reduce the use of implants as much as possible in order to minimize hardware complications. Screws still can be used, even in the usually unfixed Reverdin-Isham or Akin procedures, if the surgeon is more comfortable with fixation. If the osteotomies are not fixed, stabilization by proper postoperative dressing plays a crucial role to prevent secondary displacement. Much more than in open procedures, meticulous dressing plays an important role in the success of the operation, so the patient must continue to attend the same practice for treatment to accomplish the goals of surgery. The dressing has to be done by the surgeon or by carefully selected and well-trained employees that are familiar with the method.

If secondary displacement still develops, it must be watched and controlled carefully. The need for revision depends on the patient's problems in daily life. Often it is only a matter of radiological changes that remain unnoticed by the patient and do not affect daily life. In these cases, which represent most cases, no surgical action is needed. Otherwise, surgical repositioning and usually fixation are needed.

Overcorrection

From time to time overcorrection can be found, most likely in unfixed Akin osteotomies. Akin procedure sometimes can be performed as a complete osteotomy to correct malrotation of the big toe (discussed earlier). Even then it does not necessarily have to be fixed by hardware but can instead be taped accurately for the following 6 weeks. In the first 2 weeks, this should be done in the surgeon's own practice, afterward in can be handed over to the patient if the patient is well instructed. However, sometimes patients do too much and tape the toe into varus position. This problem can be avoided by fixing the Akin with a screw just as in the open procedure. This technique also prevents dorsal deviation in the osteotomy, which is also seen from time to time. If these results from inaccurate taping are detected not later than 6 weeks after the operation, the toe often is flexible enough to tape the varus back into the desired position. If the position is already fixed postoperatively or patients come to see the surgeon after an operation years ago, it must be corrected by surgical means. This correction can be done with an MIS or open technique.

For correction of varus malposition that is not too great, a reversed Akin procedure can be used, either fixed by screw or just followed by proper dressing.

Transfer Metatarsalgia

The treatment of transfer metatarsalgia starts with the wearing of insoles to reduce pressure under the aching metatarsal heads and also physiotherapy, especially in cases of shortening of the gastrocnemius muscles. If pain persists, surgical treatment is necessary depending on the underlying cause.

If the cause is a shortening of the first metatarsal/overlength of the lesser rays, a percutaneous distal metatarsal metaphyseal osteotomy (DMMO) of the symptomatic metatarsals is an adequate solution to the problem. In contrast to the Weil osteotomy in open surgery, the DMMO is done extra-articularly to avoid stiffness in the MTP joints. Patients are mobilized with immediate full weight bearing in order to achieve a proper realignment of the metatarsals under weight-bearing conditions.[25,26] It is important never to do only a single metatarsal. In order to prevent transfer metatarsalgia of the next ray, the correction of at least 2 must always be done, and, depending on the clinical findings, 3 rays at a time may be done.

If the reason for transfer metatarsalgia is a lack of plantarization of the first metatarsal, a plantarizing reoperation is necessary.

SUMMARY

In recent years, MIS has proved to be as safe and effective in the treatment of hallux valgus as open surgery.

In general, the same problems and complications can be observed as in open techniques. In addition, some MIS-specific complications, such as thermal lesions of the skin by the running burr, may be found. The ways of dealing with complications follow the same considerations as are known from open surgery: at first, surgeons should go for nonoperative solutions to the problem. If this is not possible, an operation must be considered. The strategy for an operative procedure, percutaneously or via open technique, depends on the specific case and the experience of the surgeon.

It has to be stressed that, in order to avoid complications, intensive training is essential. This training includes specialized MIS courses with cadaveric training and visiting experienced colleges to profit from their experience.

DISCLOSURE

The author is a consultant for MAXXOS Medical GmbH.

REFERENCES

1. Lee KT, Park YU. Deceptions in Hallux valgus: what to look for to limit failures. Foot Ankle Clin 2014;19:361–70.
2. Baravarian B, Ben-Ad R. Revision Hallux valgus: causes und correction options. Clin Podiatr Med Surg 2014;31:291–8.
3. Barg A, Harmer JR, Presson AP, et al. Unfavorable outcomes following surgical treatment of Hallux valgus deformity: a systematic literature review. J Bone Joint Surg Am 2018;100(18):1563–73.
4. Lagaay PM, Hamillton GA, Ford LA, et al. Rates of revision surgery using Chevron-austin osteotomy, lapidus arthrodeses and closing wedge base osteotomy for correction of hallux valgus deformity. J Foot Ankle Surg 2008;47:267–72.
5. Arbat D, Schneider LM, Schnurr C. Treatment of hallux valgus: current diagnostic testing and surgical treatment performed by german foot and ankle surgeons. Z Orthop Unfall 2018;156(2):193–9.
6. Altenberger S, Kriegelstein S, Gottschalk O, et al. The minimally invasive chevron and akin osteotomy. Oper Orthop Traumatol 2018;30(3):148–60.
7. Chan CX, Jan JZ, Chong HC, et al. Two year outcomes of minimally invasive hallux valgus surgery. Foot Ankle Surg 2019;25(2):119–26.
8. Kaufmann G, Dammerer D, Heyenbrock F. Minimally invasive versus open chevron osteotomy for hallux valgus correction: a randomized controlled trial. Int Orthop 2019;43(2):343–50.
9. Boksh K, Qasim S, Khan K, et al. A comparative study of mini-scarf versus standard scarf osteotomy for the hallux valgus correction. J Foot Ankle Surg 2018; 57(5):948–51.
10. Redfern D, Perera AM. Minimally invasive osteotomies. Foot Ankle Clin 2014; 19(2):181–9.
11. Dhukaran V, Chapman AP, Upadhyay PK. Minimally invasive forefoot surgery: a cadaveric study. Foot Ankle Int 2012;33(12):1139–44.
12. Durston A, Bahoo R, Kadambande S, et al. Minimally invasive calcaneal osteotomy: does the shannon burr endanger the neurovascular structures? A cadaveric study. J Foot Ankle Surg 2015;54(6):1062–6.

13. Bauer T, De Lavigne C, Biau D, et al. Percutaneous hallux valgus surgery: a prospective multicenter study of 189 cases. Orthop Clin North Am 2009;40:505–14.
14. Bauer T, Biau D, Lortat-Jacob A, et al. Percutaneous hallux valgus correction using the reverdin-isham osteotomy. Orthop Traumatol Surg Res 2010;96(4): 407–16.
15. Yassin M, Bowirat A, Robinson D. Percutaneous surgery of the forefoot compared with open technique – functional results, complications and patient satisfaction. Foot Ankle Surg 2020;26(2):156–62.
16. De Prado M. Complications in minimally invasive foot surgery. Fuß Sprunggelenk 2013;11:93–4.
17. Giannini S, Faldini S, Nani M. A minimally invasive technique for surgical treatment of hallux valgus: simple, effective, rapid, inexpensive (SERI). Int Orthop 2013;37(9):1805–13.
18. Redfern D, Vernois J, Legre BP. Percutaneous surgery of the forefoot. Clin Podiatr Med Surg 2015;32(3):291–332.
19. Malagelada F, Dalmau-Pastor M, Fargues B, et al. Increasing the safety of minimally invasive hallux surgery – an anatomical study introducing the clock method. Foot Ankle Surg 2018;24(1):40–4.
20. Bia A, Guerra-Pinto F, Pereira BS, et al. Percutaneous osteotomies in hallux valgus: a systematic review. J Foot Ankle Surg 2018;57(1):123–30.
21. Frigg A, Zaugg S, Maquieira G, et al. Stiffness at rate of motion of the minimally invasive chevron-akin and open scarf-akin procedures. Foot Ankle Int 2019;40(5): 515–25.
22. Severyns M, Carrret P, Bruniet-Agot L, et al. Reverdin-Isham procedure for mild or moderate hallux valgus: clinical and radiological outcomes. Muskuloskelet Surg 2019;103(2):161–6.
23. De Lavigne C, Rasmont Q, Hoang B. Percutaneous double metatarsal osteotomy for correction of severe hallux valgus deformity. Acta Orthop Belg 2011;77(4): 516–21.
24. Restuccia G, Lippi A, Sacchetti F, et al. Percutaneous hallux valgus correction: modified reverdin-isham osteotomy, preliminary results. Surg Technol Int 2017; 31:262–6.
25. Thomas M, Jordan M. Minimally invasive correction of lesser toes deformities and treatment of metatarsalgia. Oper Orthop Traumatol 2018;30(3):171–83.
26. Malhotra K, Joji N, Mordecai S, et al. Minimally invasive distal metaphyseal metatarsal osteotomy (DMMO) for symptomatic forefoot pathology - Short to medium term outcomes from a retrospective case series. Foot (Edinb) 2019;38:43–9.

Lapidus, a Percutaneous Approach

Joel Vernois, MD[a,b,]*, David Redfern, MBBS, FRCS[c,d], GRECMIP soon MIFAS[e]

KEYWORDS

- Lapidus • Percutaneous • Mini-invasive surgery • Forefoot • Hallux valgus
- Tarsometatarsal • Arthrodesis

KEY POINTS

- The percutaneous Lapidus procedure is a powerful but demanding technique.
- Its is a less aggressive procedure than open procedure.
- It is less painful, with less swelling.
- The percutaneous Lapidus procedure needs specific training.

INTRODUCTION

First ray deformity is a common pathologic condition. Different options of treatment have been described in open techniques, such as the Lapidus. First ray deformity treatments were initially described by Albrecht, but were reported by Lapidus in 1934, who gave his name to this powerful procedure.[1,2] The Lapidus is probably the most versatile procedure in foot and ankle surgery. Used in many circumstances, it offers a stable and reliable correction. Its aim is to fuse the first tarsometatarsal joint (TMT) in an adequate position. The procedure is used in different pathologic conditions, such as first TMT instability, hallux valgus deformity, flat foot deformity, and TMT arthritis. Introduced in Europe by Mariano De Prado in the 1990s and promoted by the GRECMIP since 2004, percutaneous surgery offers a large range of possible treatments. A percutaneous Lapidus procedure became a real option for patients.

No conflict of interest.
[a] Sussex Orthopaedic NHS Treatment Centre, Lewes Road, Haywards Heath, West Sussex RH16 4EY, England; [b] ICP, Clinique Blomet, 136bis rue Blomet, Paris 75015, France; [c] Montefiore Hospital, Hove, East Sussex, England; [d] London Foot and Ankle Centre, Hospital of St John and St Elizabeth, 60 Grove End Road, London NW8 9NH, England; [e] 2 rue Nègre-Vergne, Lot. Hermitage Est, Merignac 33700, France
* Corresponding author. Sussex Orthopaedic NHS Treatment Centre, Lewes Road, Haywards Heath, West Sussex RH16 4EY, England.
E-mail address: joel.vernois@sfr.fr

SURGICAL TECHNIQUES
Equipment

Beaver blade

Burr: Wedge, 12 × 3 mm, and a Shannon, 20 × 2 mm and 20 × 3 mm

K-wire: 2 K-wires of 2-mm diameter

Screws: 2 to 3 screws of 4 mm

Driver: Must have high torque so it can be used with a low speed. High speed is responsible for thermal injury to the skin and the bone. Irrigation would be also preferable for cooling the burr.

C-arm: Mini, rather than large, is easier to maneuver.

Tourniquet: It is a surgeon choice. Blood is an excellent cooling system. If a tourniquet is used, irrigation is highly recommended.

Anesthesia

Regional ankle block or general anesthesia depends on the expertise of the anesthetist. A single dose of antibiotics is suggested as per local guidelines.

Positioning

The patient is positioned supine with the foot overhanging the end of the table. The C-arm is positioned under the foot for an immediate control of the procedure.

THE TECHNIQUE

The surgery is performed under radiograph control. The TMT is localized with fluoroscopy.

To avoid excessive shortening, 2 K-wires are placed vertically on both sides of the joint (**Fig. 1**). Their positions and directions would dictate the amount of correction and the potential shortening. If lowering of the head is necessary, the K-wires would be divergent (**Fig. 2**). The position of the K-wire is very important. It will determine the resection and the correction. It is recommended to go through the sole of the foot and hold the K-wire with a clip.

A medial approach, 1 cm, is realized at the level of the TMT joint. The 20 × 2-mm burr is introduced in the joint and run parallel to the K-wire. It is important to release the medial cuneometatarsal ligament to open and mobilize the joint. The plantar part of the joint must be carefully prepared. If needed, the wedge burr or the 20 × 3-mm Shannon burr can be used. The osteotomy starts at the level of the cuneiform bone, perpendicular to the second metatarsal along the proximal K-wire. The resection must be minimal. As soon as this first stage is performed, the joint becomes

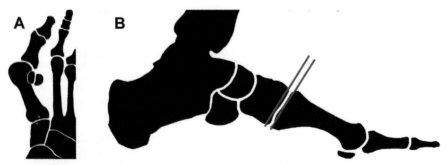

Fig. 1. (*A, B*) Position of the parallel K-wire at the level of the cuneometatarsal joint.

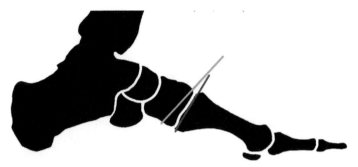

Fig. 2. Divergent K-wire.

particularly mobile. The deformity can be corrected. The second stage is the osteotomy of the base of M1. It must be parallel to the first stage cut with the first metatarsal in a correct position. The distal K-wire guarantees minimal resection (**Fig. 3**).

Once the correction is completed, the bones are then fixed with 2 or 3 crossed screws (**Fig. 4**). The first screw is positioned horizontal from distal to proximal and medial to lateral, and the second screw is positioned vertical from proximal to distal. If instability between the first and the second cuneiform is noted, then a third screw is positioned between the first and second metatarsal (**Fig. 5**).

The wounds are closed with absorbable sutures.

Postoperative Care

- The dressing is left undisturbed for 2 weeks.
- The foot is kept elevated.
- An orthopedic heel shoe is required for 6 weeks with the help of crutches.

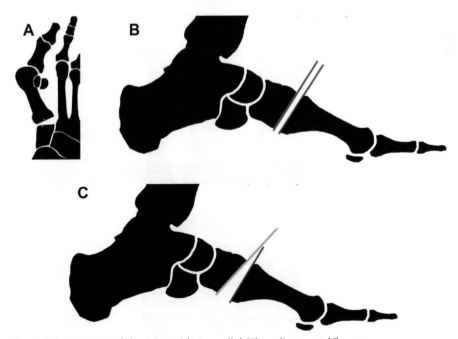

Fig. 3. (*A*) Resection of the joint with 2 parallel (*B*) or divergent (*C*) cuts.

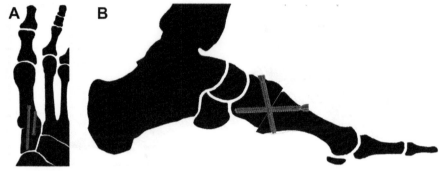

Fig. 4. Fixation with 2 cross-screws. AP view (*A*), Lateral view (*B*).

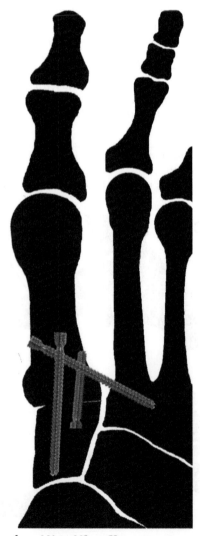

Fig. 5. An additional screw from M1 to M2 or C2.

- At 6 weeks' follow-up, radiographs are requested. If the healing is correct, the patient can wear normal shoes.
- Impact on the forefoot is authorized from 3 months.

Indication

- Flat feet
- Arthritis
- Hallux valgus

RESULTS

Seventy feet treated with a percutaneous Lapidus were followed and reviewed. All cases have been performed by a single surgeon. All the patients have been reviewed at 2 and 6 weeks and then at 3 and 6 months postoperatively both clinically and radiologically. An Akin osteotomy has been routinely performed. No additional distal osteotomy has been requested. The procedure has been used for a flat foot correction on 10 occasions.

The average age of the population was 69 years.

The satisfaction rate was good and excellent for 95% of the patients.

Four patients presented a nonunion.

No metatarsalgia transfers and no infections have been reported.

DISCUSSION

Lapidus has been used since 1934 for the treatment of hallux valgus. A powerful technique, Lapidus allows a great deal of correction, but there are some pitfalls that must be avoided. The position and the orientation of the cut are essential. This lies in the position of the K-wires. If too medial, too much bone may be removed; too lateral, and not enough is removed to obtain the correction. If not close enough to the joint, then too much bone may also be removed. An excess of shortening may be responsible of secondary metatarsalgia even with the lowering of the head. That is why an index minus is probably not a good indication for a Lapidus. Parallel to each other, the metatarsal will not be lowering. Divergent, the metatarsal head will be lowering depending on the angulation between the 2 K-wires. The quality of the correction depends on the release of the TMT joint and the removal of the debris left in the joint particularly on the plantar part.

A lateral release at the metatarsophalangeal joint is not systematic for the authors except if a retraction of the capsule is present.

Since the authors promoted percutaneous surgery, they have heard many concerns about the safety of using a burr. If the technique is not safe and reproducible, it will fail. The authors use a medial approach to prepare the joint and recommend an "extensive" approach of 8 to 10 mm. The burr is introduced in the joint and must stay in the joint. The rotation and the size of the portal avoid any burning on the skin. A cooling system can be associated particularly if a tourniquet is inflated.

The structures at risk are on the dorsal part of the joint and lateral distal part.[3,4] Because the burr stays in the joint, any damage would be a surprise and a surgical mistake because the burr's spinning should be stopped as soon as the dorsal or plantar capsule is reached. The position of the K-wire "guide" must be carefully decided to avoid a lesion of the superficial peroneal nerve or the dorsal-medial artery. A medial position to the tendon extensor would be preferable. In the authors' experience, no injury has been report at the level of the TMT joint. The fixation is realized with 2 cross-screws, and if necessary, an intermetatarsal third screw. The authors recommend a distal horizontal screw positioned 3 to 4 cm distal to the joint line on the lateral side of the extensor tendon. The proximal screw would be inserted through a dorsal-lateral 5-mm approach to the extensor tendon. The need of a third screw occurs when instability between first and second cuneiform bone is revealed. The squeeze test is helpful to determine this need.[5]

The average age of the authors' population is older than the usual publication[6-9] because the authors prefer to perform a basal osteotomy on the younger population.

Surgeons have always tried to optimize the recovery and minimize their approach. Michels and Lui[10,11] presented an interesting arthroscopic Lapidus procedure, but in the authors' hands, it seems to be a longer procedure with no advantage compared with the percutaneous technique. As for Michels' and other techniques, an additional distal osteotomy is needed.

The authors' only concern raised is the shortening of the first ray. Even if no metatarsalgia has been reported, a longer follow-up may shed more light on this.

SUMMARY

Lapidus percutaneous correction is a very interesting procedure, but excessive shortening remains a concern and could potentially result in metatarsalgia.

REFERENCES

1. Lapidus PW. A quarter of a century of experience with the operative correction of the metatarsus varus primus in hallux valgus. Bull Hosp Joint Dis 1956;17(2): 404-21.
2. Lapidus PW. The author's bunion operation from 1931 to 1959. Clin Orthop 1960; 16:119-35.
3. So E, Van Dyke B, McGann MR, et al. Structures at risk from an intermetatarsal screw for Lapidus bunionectomy: a cadaveric study. J Foot Ankle Surg 2019; 58(1):62-5.
4. Lehtonen E, Patel H, Lee S, et al. Neurovascular structures at risk with percutaneous fixation in tarsometatarsal fusion: a cadaveric study. Foot (Edinb) 2019; 41:19-23.
5. Vernois J, Redfern DJ. Percutaneous surgery for severe hallux valgus. Foot Ankle Clin 2016;21(3):479-93.
6. Boffeli TJ, Mahoney KJ. Intraoperative simulated weightbearing lateral foot imaging: the clinical utility and ability to predict sagittal plane position of the first ray in lapidus fusion. J Foot Ankle Surg 2016;55(6):1158-63.
7. Ellington JK, Myerson MS, Coetzee JC, et al. The use of the Lapidus procedure for recurrent hallux valgus. Foot Ankle Int 2011;32(7):674-80.
8. Jagadale VS, Thomas RL. A clinicoradiological and functional evaluation of Lapidus surgery for moderate to severe bunion deformity shows excellent stable correction and high long-term patient satisfaction. Foot Ankle Spec 2019. https://doi.org/10.1177/1938640019890716. 1938640019890716.
9. Popelka S, Vavrík P, Hromádka R, et al. Our results of the Lapidus procedure in patients with hallux valgus deformity. Acta Chir Orthop Traumatol Cech 2008; 75(4):271-6 [in Czech].
10. Lui TH, Chan KB, Chow HT, et al. Arthroscopy-assisted correction of hallux valgus deformity. Arthroscopy 2008;24(8):875-80.
11. Michels F, Guillo S, de Lavigne C, et al. The arthroscopic Lapidus procedure. Foot Ankle Surg 2011;17(1):25-8.

The Windswept Foot: Dealing with Metatarsus Adductus and Toe Valgus

Anna-Kathrin Leucht, MD[a,b,1],
Alastair Younger, MB ChB, MSc, ChM, FRCSC[a,*],
Andrea Veljkovic, MD, MPH(Harvard), BComm, FRCSC[a],
Anthony Perera, MBChB, MRCS, MFSEM (RCP & SI), FRCS (Orth)[c]

KEYWORDS

- Metatarsus adductus • Windswept deformity • Toe valgus • Minimal invasive
- Forefoot deformity

KEY POINTS

- The deformity correction of a windswept foot (hallux valgus deformity in a setting of a metatarsus adductus and toe valgus) is challenging and no clear consensus is available regarding the optimal treatment.
- Depending on the severity of the deformity, open or percutaneous distal metatarsal osteotomies, percutaneous proximal metatarsal osteotomies, percutaneous tarsometatarsal fusion, which can be performed percutaneously or using a hybrid technique, may be required.
- To correct the lesser toe deformities, additional percutaneous techniques adjusted to the specific toe position are needed.

INTRODUCTION

Metatarsus adductus is a congenital, uniplanar deformity in the transverse plane, which is defined by adduction of the metatarsals in relation to the tarsus with a neutral hindfoot.[1–3] The deformity is centered at the Lisfranc joint line[4] and, as such, is a solely 1-level forefoot deformity. It is differentiated from more complex congenital foot deformity with metatarsus adductus including screwfoot deformity, which is defined by additional midfoot abduction and hindfoot valgus or clubfoot with heel equinus and varus.

[a] Footbridge Clinic, Unit 221, 181 Keefer Place, Vancouver, British Columbia V6B 6C1, Canada; [b] Department of Orthopaedics and Traumatology, Cantonal Hospital of Winterthur, Switzerland; [c] University Hospital of Wales Llandough, University Hospital of Wales Cardiff, Spire Cardiff Hospital, Croescadaran Road, Cardiff, Wales CF23 8XL, UK
[1] Present address: Büchnerstrasse 1, 8996 Zürich, Switzerland
* Corresponding author.
E-mail address: alastair.stephen.younger@gmail.com

Foot Ankle Clin N Am 25 (2020) 413–424
https://doi.org/10.1016/j.fcl.2020.05.005
1083-7515/20/© 2020 Elsevier Inc. All rights reserved.

The metatarsus adductus is one of the most common foot deformities, with an incidence of 1 to 2 per 1000 births.[5–8] The cause of metatarsus adductus is not completely understood, but an association with increased intrauterine pressure, supported by increased incidence in twin gestation, is assumed. Other theories include osseous abnormalities and/or atypical muscle attachments.[9,10]

Metatarsus adductus seems to predispose to the development of hallux valgus.[11–13] In several studies, a prevalence of metatarsus adductus in 22% to 35% of patients with hallux valgus deformity has been found,[1,14,15] and patients with metatarsus adductus have a 3.5 times higher chance to develop a hallux valgus deformity.[1] Furthermore, lesser toe deformity, such as lateral windswept toes, are commonly found in association with metatarsus adductus.

BIOMECHANICS

The adducted forefoot leads to valgus deforming forces at the level of the first metatarsophalangeal (MTP) joint in normal shoe wear.[16] In long-standing deformity, the adduction of the metatarsals subsequently leads to failure of the medial-sided capsular complex of the MTP joints, including the medial collateral, whereas the lateral side tightens. Once the medial capsule is incompetent, the deformity progresses. The adductor provides the main deforming force on the hallux, but displacement by the extensor hallucis longus additionally contributes to the valgus deformity with its eccentric pull. A similar pathomechanism is applicable for the lesser MTP joints. As the angular deformity increases, the sagittal joint stability subsequently decreases, which triggers lesser toe deformities such as hammer toes in combination with the valgus windswept toes.

RELEVANCE

The recognition of a metatarsus adductus deformity in patients with hallux valgus is crucial and it affects the outcome of surgical correction. Because of the adduction of the lesser metatarsals, the hallux valgus deformity is prone to be underestimated because of a reduced intermetatarsal angle (IMA). Therefore, failing to notice the metatarsus adductus deformity can lead to an undercorrection of the hallux valgus. In addition, the adduction of the second metatarsal reduces the intermetatarsal interval, which is needed for the lateral translation of the head in distal osteotomies and thus diminishes the correction potential of these.

Aiyer and colleagues[14] found a significantly higher radiographic recurrence of hallux valgus in the setting of a metatarsus adductus (28.9%) compared with the control group (15.2%). In line with the previously mentioned difficulties of distal osteotomies in metatarsus adductus, the risk of recurrence in less severe metatarsus adductus was higher (80%) compared with the group with severe deformity. Most of the moderate deformities were corrected with chevron osteotomies alone, whereas the severe deformities without recurrence were treated with more aggressive corrections, including realignment of the lesser metatarsals.

Higher Rate of Lesser Metatarsophalangeal Deformity

Metatarsus adductus might be combined with lesser toe deformities of any kind. In severe metatarsus adductus, a prevalence of 53% of lesser toe deformity was found in a study by Aiyer and colleagues.[17] In our clinical experience, the rate of toe deformity associated with severe metatarsus adductus might even be higher than 53%, especially in the older patient group. In lower degrees of metatarsus adductus, the lesser toe deformity might not be as obvious.

The lesser toe deformity, in particular the valgus windswept deformity, has an impact on the surgical strategy as well. If the correction is only focused on the hallux valgus deformity, a gap between the first and second toe will be created, which will lead to a loss of the buttress effect of the second toe and might cause a recurrence of the hallux valgus.[18]

Fifth Metatarsal Fracture at the Metadiaphyseal Junction

The altered anatomy of the foot in metatarsus adductus leads to a lateral column overload, with increased peak pressure at the metadiaphyseal junction of the fifth metatarsal. Compared with the mobile fifth metatarsal head, the base of the fifth metatarsal has firm capsular attachments to the fourth metatarsal and the cuboid. In addition, the peroneus brevis and the plantar fascia attach at the base of the fifth metatarsal. With loading of the lateral column, a peak stress culminates at the fulcrum, the metadiaphyseal junction.[19,20] Any excessive load directed to the metadiaphyseal junction of the fifth metatarsal may result in a Jones-type fracture, as seen in athletes with repeated cutting and pivoting motions, who are notably predisposed to Jones fractures because of the increased vertical and mediolateral forces to the lateral aspect of the foot. Therefore, it is not surprising that a correlation between metatarsus adductus and the incidence of Jones fracture was found, and to our knowledge was first described in 1999 by Theodorou and colleagues.[21] In 1 retrospective study, the metatarsus adductus angle (MAA) was measured in a group of patient with metadiaphyseal fractures of the fifth metatarsal. The analysis revealed a significant higher mean MAA in the Jones fracture group ($20.22°$) compared with an asymptomatic control group ($14.27°$).[22] The same group showed a strong positive correlation between the severity of metatarsus adductus and bone healing time; patients with higher MAA showed a longer time to complete bony union of the Jones-type fracture.[23]

The association of proximal diaphyseal stress fractures of the fifth metatarsal with metatarsus adductus was additionally investigated by Warmelink,[24] who again found a significant higher mean MAA of $26.35°$ in the stress fracture group compared with the control group.

PHYSICAL EXAMINATION

In the clinical examination, the foot appears C shaped because of a concave medial border and convex lateral border with a prominent base of the fifth metatarsal bone. The hindfoot shows a normal alignment or slight valgus. According to La Reaux and Lee,[1] a number of criteria must coincide to diagnose a metatarsus adductus: a high arch, adduction and inversion of the forefoot, a prominent lateral border, and the inability to abduct the foot beyond the midline to an increased rigidity.

The distinctive signs mentioned earlier are more likely to be found in pediatric patients, and might be less pronounced in adults with a metatarsus adductus. Adults with metatarsus adductus tend to present with a hallux valgus and lesser toe deformity. The latter includes valgus windswept deformity, hammer toes, or a combination of both.

Additional typical symptoms of patients with metatarsus adductus are metatarsalgia with painful callus over the plantar aspect of the second and third plantar head, as well as skin irritation over the medial eminence in the setting of a hallux valgus.

IMAGING

Standardized weight-bearing radiographs are required to assess the metatarsus adductus deformity. On radiograph, excessive adduction of all metatarsals at the level of the Lisfranc joint is visible. Typically, the second and third metatarsals present with a higher degree of medial deviation than the fourth and fifth metatarsals. In addition, a distinctive overlapping of the base of the metatarsals can be recognized. Care must also be taken to ensure that the patient is loading the medial border of the foot on the standing radiograph because varus alignment of the foot during the imaging makes the foot seem adductus.

Several different MAAs are described in the literature to determine the grade of deformity. Two of them are frequently used in recent literature: the Sgarlato method and the Engel angle.

In the Sgarlato method, the MAA is defined as the angle between the longitudinal axis of the metatarsus (longitudinal axis of the second metatarsal) and the longitudinal axis of the lesser tarsus. To find the longitudinal axis of the lesser tarsus, a line from the most medial aspect of the first metatarsal to the talonavicular joint and a line from the most lateral aspect of the fourth metatarsal-cuboid and the calcaneocuboid joint is drawn. A connection line between the midpoints of these 2 lines defines the transverse axis of the lesser tarsus, and a perpendicular line to this depicts the longitudinal axis of the lesser tarsus (**Fig. 1**).[25] A modified version of the Sgarlato angle uses the lateral aspect of the fifth metatarsal-cuboid and calcaneocuboid joint as landmarks for the lateral line. The Engel angle uses a line that bisects the middle cuneiform to represent the longitudinal axis of the lesser tarsus, which is a simplified, convenient version to measure the MAA.[26] However, note that the Engel angle is consistently 3° greater than the MAA of Sgarlato.[27] Applying the traditional method to quantify the MAA, it is possible to distinguish between a mild (15°–20°), moderate (21°–25°), and a severe (>25°) metatarsus adductus deformity.[28] The normal range of the MAA is defined as 8° to 14°.[29]

The Sgarlato method showed the highest interobserver and intraobserver reliability in addition to showing a significant a positive correlation between hallux valgus angle and MAA in a study by Dawoodi and Perera.[30]

The IMA is frequently used for preoperative planning in hallux valgus deformity correction. In metatarsus adductus, the IMA is low because of the adduction of the second metatarsal and therefore the deformity is underestimated. A formula was recommended by Yu and Dinapoli[28] to determine the true IMA: true IMA = IMA + (MAA − 15°). The angle 15° represents the lowest MAA to be classified as metatarsus adductus and therefore the formula still bears some risk of underestimating the IMA.

Furthermore, lesser toe deformities can be assessed, and hammer or claw toe and the typical lesser toe valgus deformity (which results in a windswept deformity) differentiated, using standardized radiographs.

A computed tomography (CT) can help to distinguish the amount of degenerative changes present at the Lisfranc joint line and therefore assist in the decision making between possible surgical treatment options. In severe metatarsus adductus, where a correction of the alignment of the second and third metatarsals is necessary and osteoarthritis is present, the correction of the deformity can be accomplished by a 1-3 tarsometatarsal (TMT) fusion.

Metatarsus adductus has, to our knowledge, not been studied in weight-bearing CT scans, and this might be of interest for further studies.

TREATMENT: NONOPERATIVE

Nonoperative treatment should be exhausted before surgical management. Nonoperative treatment includes customized orthotics and modification of shoe wear with wide

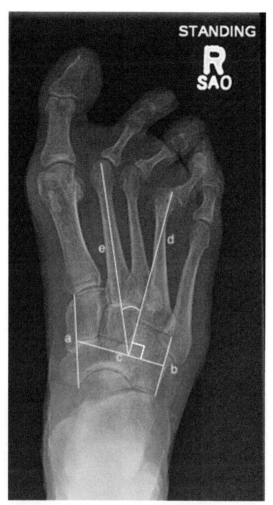

Fig. 1. Sgarlato metatarsus adductus angle. Line a extends between the most medial aspect of the first tarsometatarsal (TMT) joint and the talonavicular joint. Line b extends between the most lateral aspect of the fourth TMT joint and the calcaneocuboid joint. Line c is drawn from the midpoints of line a and b, a perpendicular line d to line c represents the longitudinal axis of the lesser tarsus, whereas line e represents the longitudinal axis of the second metatarsal. The angle between line e and d is the traditional Sgarlato angle.

toe box. In lesser toe deformities, silicon sleeves and toe spacers prevent painful calluses. Regular stretching exercises of the gastrocnemius reduce forefoot pressure in patients in whom metatarsalgia is a major component.

TREATMENT: OPERATIVE

The treatment of hallux valgus and subsequent lesser toe deformity in metatarsus adductus is challenging. There is no clear evidence for which procedure is the optimum regarding outcome, recurrence, and complications. This article presents different minimally invasive and hybrid surgical options to address this deformity depending on the severity of the metatarsus adductus.

1. Hallux valgus correction plus or minus metatarsus adductus correction
   A. Percutaneous first TMT fusion plus or minus distal metatarsal osteotomies (percutaneous or open): In mild metatarsus adductus, the hallux valgus deformity can be addressed with a percutaneous Lapidus procedure alone. The percutaneous Lapidus procedure is our standard procedure for the correction of hallux valgus deformities and is done by a percutaneous lateral release of the first MTP joint, a percutaneous resection of the medial eminence, followed by a preparation of the first TMT joint with the 2 × 12 burr. The residual cartilage is debrided under direct visualization (2.9-mm scope) with either the burr or the shaver. After reduction of the first metatarsal with correct rotation, abduction, and plantar flexion, we stabilize the joint with 3 percutaneous screws and 1 intermetatarsal screw from the base of the first to the base of the second metatarsal. A clinical example is shown in **Fig. 2**; in this case, the decision against an additional proximal osteotomy of the second and third metatarsal was made intraoperatively. In addition, the typical screw position for the percutaneous Lapidus procedure is shown.If symptomatic windswept toes are present, distal metatarsal osteotomies, either percutaneous or Weil osteotomies (as shown in **Fig. 3**), can be added. In our opinion, screw fixation leads to a more predictable outcome, reducing the risk of any secondary rotational change during the healing period, as seen in **Fig. 4**.Reviewing the outcome of the case in **Fig. 4**, a

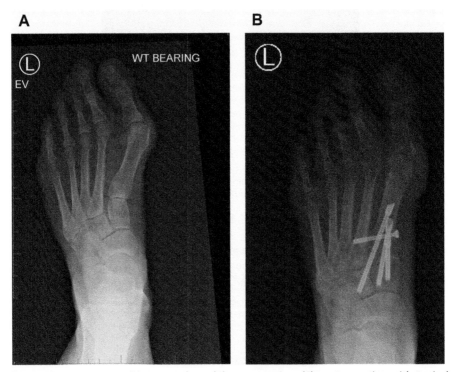

Fig. 2. Percutaneous Lapidus procedure: (*A*) preoperative, (*B*) postoperative with typical screw position.

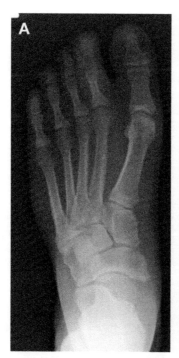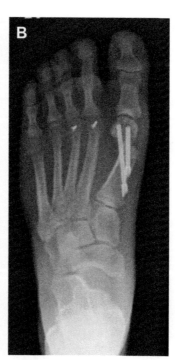

Fig. 3. Percutaneous chevron osteotomy with additional open Weil osteotomies of the second and third metatarsals: (*A*) preoperative, (*B*) postoperative.

proximal metatarsal osteotomy to realign the eccentric pull of the tendons would have been necessary.

B. Percutaneous chevron osteotomy plus or minus distal metatarsal osteotomies (percutaneous or open): In **Fig. 3**, a percutaneous chevron osteotomy is presented in a setting of a mild metatarsus adductus. This procedure is performed as an extra-articular V-shaped osteotomy, which is directed 10° plantarly to avoid elevation and 10° distally to maintain the first metatarsal length as described by Vernois and Redfern.[31,32] The fixation was obtained with 2 screws. In this case, open Weil osteotomies were added to address the lesser toe deformities.

C. Percutaneous first to third TMT fusion with correction of metatarsus adductus: In patients with hallux valgus and concomitant second and third TMT arthritis and severe metatarsus adductus, the correction of the deviation of the lesser metatarsals can be achieved with an arthrodesis of the second and third TMT joints in a realigned position along with the Lapidus procedure for the hallux valgus. This procedure can be performed percutaneously as well, using the burr for the preparation of the second and third TMT joints and the scope to control the complete debridement. The fixation is accomplished with percutaneous screws crossing the TMT joints (**Fig. 5**, open correction; **Fig. 6**, clinical example of percutaneous 1–3 TMT fusion). By achieving a structural alignment of the metatarsals at the TMT level, a centric pull of the extrinsic and intrinsic muscles is restored and leads to improved position of the valgus toe deformity at the level of the MTP joint.

D. Percutaneous proximal osteotomies and percutaneous first TMT fusion: In severe metatarsus adductus and hallux valgus but absence of degenerative

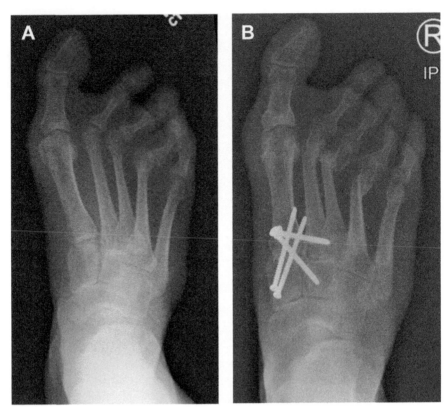

Fig. 4. Residual windswept deformity of lesser toes after surgical correction with Lapidus procedure and distal metatarsal metaphyseal osteotomies (DMMOs): (*A*) preoperative, (*B*) postoperative. Percutaneous distal metatarsal osteotomies allow lateral displacement of the lesser metatarsal heads, but it is hard to control the metatarsal heads and toes remaining in valgus. For this reason, proximal osteotomies or fusions may be a better choice.

changes over the TMT joint, the correction of the lesser metatarsals can be performed with minimal invasive, lateral closing wedge osteotomies. These osteotomies need temporary Kirschner wire fixation or screw fixation to heal successfully. The additional hallux valgus deformity can be addressed with the percutaneous Lapidus procedure, as mentioned earlier. The minimally invasive surgery (MIS) closing wedge osteotomies are shown in a complex case of Dr Anthony Perera in **Fig. 7**, where a revision of a hallux valgus correction was achieved with a proximal closing wedge of the first metatarsal (MT1) and an MIS first MTP fusion.

E. Percutaneous first MTP fusion: A solid alternative surgical option to the percutaneous Lapidus procedure mentioned earlier to correct a hallux valgus in a metatarsus adductus is a first MTP fusion. The fusion does not noticeably correct the broad forefoot, which must be explained to the patient to set correct expectations, but it rules out hallux valgus recurrence, stabilizes the first ray, and reestablishes weight bearing over the medial column.[33,34]The percutaneous technique in our hands consists of complete resection of the cartilage with the 2 × 12-mm Shannon burr; first MTP joint arthroscopy to debride any remaining cartilage

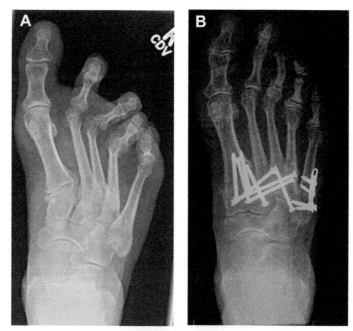

Fig. 5. First to third TMT fusion with correction of metatarsus adductus, open correction, with additional fifth ray and phalangeal osteotomies: (A) preoperative, (B) postoperative.

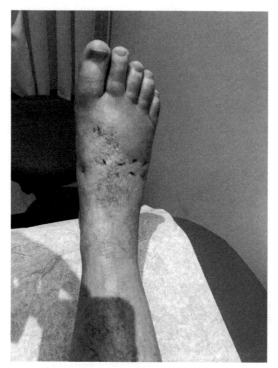

Fig. 6. Clinical example of percutaneous 1 to 3 TMT fusion.

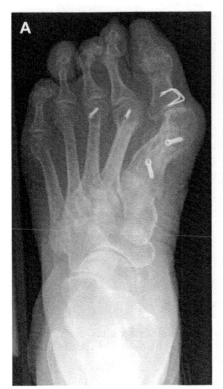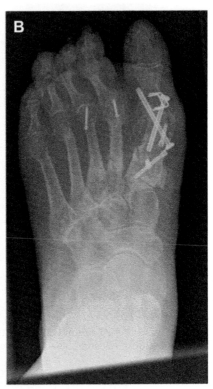

Fig. 7. Complex case with revision of hallux valgus correction with proximal MIS closing wedge osteotomies, screw fixation of the first metatarsal (MT1), temporary Kirschner wire fixation of MT2 and MT3, DMMO of MT4, and MIS first MTP fusion: (*A*) preoperative, (*B*) postoperative. (*Courtesy of* A. Perera, MD, MBChB, MRCS, MFSEM, (RCP & SI), FRCS (Orth), Cardiff, UK.)

areas with the shaver and to irrigate the joint; followed by percutaneous fixation with 2 to 3 crossing, cannulated headless compression screws.

2. Treatment of the windswept lesser toes

As already mentioned, the realignment of the lesser metatarsal results in an optimized pull of the tendons at the MTP joints and reduction of the toe deformity.

Nevertheless, in long-standing, rigid deformities, additional minimal invasive procedures to correct the lesser toe deformities are necessary. These procedures include percutaneous lesser MTP releases of the lateral and dorsal capsule. Depending on the toe deformity, percutaneous basal proximal phalangeal osteotomies performed as medial closing wedge procedures for valgus deformity or plantar closing wedge for hammer toes are added in conjunction with tendon releases.

Basal fifth TMT osteotomy to release the tension on the intermetatarsal ligament.

On occasion in patients with metatarsus adductus, the fifth ray is mobile and laterally deviated. This condition places tension on the plantar plates of the lesser MTP joints and increases the valgus alignment of the lesser toes. To prevent the lateral pull of the lesser rays and narrow the foot to improve shoe wear, a percutaneous fifth metatarsal osteotomy may be required.

SUMMARY

Depending on the severity of the metatarsus adductus, the hallux valgus deformity can either be addressed alone with a percutaneous Lapidus procedure in our hands, or a multilevel surgical correction can be requested adjusted to the deformity. These deformity corrections can be performed percutaneously, demanding a thorough understanding of the anatomy and a precise surgical technique to result in a good outcome and avoid complications.

DISCLOSURE

A-K. Leucht and A. Veljkovic have nothing to disclose. A. Younger and A. Perera consult with Wright medical.

REFERENCES

1. La Reaux RL, Lee BR. Metatarsus adductus and hallux abducto valgus: their correlation. J Foot Surg 1987;26(4):304–8.
2. Rothbart BA. Metatarsus adductus and its clinical significance. J Am Podiatry Assoc 1972;62(5):187–90.
3. Root ML, Orien WP, Weed JH. Normal and abnormal function of the foot. Los Angeles: Clinical Biomechanics Corporation; 1977.
4. Heyman CH, Herndon CH, Strong JM. Mobilization of the tarsometatarsal and intermetatarsal joints for the correction of resistant adduction of the fore part of the foot in congenital club-foot or congenital metatarsus varus. J Bone Joint Surg Am 1958;40-A(2):299–309 [discussion: 309–1].
5. Wynne-Davies R. Family Studies and the Cause of Congenital Club Foot. Talipes equinovarus, talipes calcaneo-valgus and metatarsus varus. J Bone Joint Surg Br 1964;46:445–63.
6. Tax HR, Albright T. Metatarsus adducto varus: a simplified approach to treatment. J Am Podiatry Assoc 1978;68(5):331–8.
7. Tax HR. Podopediatrics. Philadelphia: Williams & Wilkins; 1985.
8. Dietz FR. Intoeing–fact, fiction and opinion. Am Fam Physician 1994;50(6): 1249–59, 1262–4.
9. Morcuende JA, Ponseti IV. Congenital metatarsus adductus in early human fetal development: a histologic study. Clin Orthop Relat Res 1996;(333):261–6.
10. Peabody CM. F. Congenital metatarsus varus. J Bone Joint Surg 1933;(15): 171–89.
11. Houghton GR, Dickson RA. Hallux valgus in the younger patient: the structural abnormality. J Bone Joint Surg Br 1979;61-B(2):176–7.
12. Mann RA, Coughlin MJ. Hallux valgus–etiology, anatomy, treatment and surgical considerations. Clin Orthop Relat Res 1981;(157):31–41.
13. Reimann I, Werner HH. Congenital metatarsus varus. A suggestion for a possible mechanism and relation to other foot deformities. Clin Orthop Relat Res 1975; 110:223–6.
14. Aiyer AA, Shariff R, Ying L, et al. Prevalence of metatarsus adductus in patients undergoing hallux valgus surgery. Foot Ankle Int 2014;35(12):1292–7.
15. Coughlin MJ. Roger A. Mann Award. Juvenile hallux valgus: etiology and treatment. Foot Ankle Int 1995;16(11):682–97.
16. Coughlin MJ, Mann RA. The pathophysiology of the juvenile bunion. Instr Course Lect 1987;36:123–36.

17. Aiyer A, Shub J, Shariff R, et al. Radiographic recurrence of deformity after hallux valgus surgery in patients with metatarsus adductus. Foot Ankle Int 2016;37(2): 165–71.
18. Kilmartin TE, O'Kane C. Correction of valgus second toe by closing wedge osteotomy of the proximal phalanx. Foot Ankle Int 2007;28(12):1260–4.
19. Wright RW, Fischer DA, Shively RA, et al. Refracture of proximal fifth metatarsal (Jones) fracture after intramedullary screw fixation in athletes. Am J Sports Med 2000;28(5):732–6.
20. Kavanaugh JH, Brower TD, Mann RV. The Jones fracture revisited. J Bone Joint Surg Am 1978;60(6):776–82.
21. Theodorou DJ, Theodorou SJ, Boutin RD, et al. Stress fractures of the lateral metatarsal bones in metatarsus adductus foot deformity: a previously unrecognized association. Skeletal Radiol 1999;28(12):679–84.
22. Yoho RM, Carrington S, Dix B, et al. The association of metatarsus adductus to the proximal fifth metatarsal Jones fracture. J Foot Ankle Surg 2012;51(6):739–42.
23. Yoho RM, Vardaxis V, Dikis J. A retrospective review of the effect of metatarsus adductus on healing time in the fifth metatarsal jones fracture. Foot (Edinb). 2015;25(4):215–9.
24. Wamelink KE, Marcoux JT, Walrath SM. Rare Proximal Diaphyseal Stress Fractures of the Fifth Metatarsal Associated With Metatarsus Adductus. J Foot Ankle Surg 2016;55:788.
25. Sgarlato TE, Medicine CCoP. A compendium of podiatric biomechanics. San Francisco: California College of Podiatric Medicine; 1971.
26. Engel E, Erlick N, Krems I. A simplified metatarsus adductus angle. J Am Podiatry Assoc 1983;73(12):620–8.
27. Thomas JL, Kunkel MW, Lopez R, et al. Radiographic values of the adult foot in a standardized population. J Foot Ankle Surg 2006;45(1):3–12.
28. Yu GD, DiNapoli R. Surgical management of hallux abductovalgus with concomitant metatarsus adductus. In: McGlamry E, editor. Reconstructive surgery of the foot and leg. Tucker (GA): Podiatry institute publishing; 1989. p. 262–8.
29. Weissman S. Biomechanically acquired foot types. In: SD W, editor. Radiology of the foot. Baltimore: Williams and Wilkins; 1989. p. 66–90.
30. Dawoodi AI, Perera A. Reliability of metatarsus adductus angle and correlation with hallux valgus. Foot Ankle Surg 2012;18(3):180–6.
31. Redfern D, Vernois J, Legre BP. Percutaneous Surgery of the Forefoot. Clin Podiatr Med Surg 2015;32(3):291–332.
32. Vernois J, Redfern DJ. Percutaneous Surgery for Severe Hallux Valgus. Foot Ankle Clin 2016;21(3):479–93.
33. Coughlin MJ, Grebing BR, Jones CP. Arthrodesis of the first metatarsophalangeal joint for idiopathic hallux valgus: intermediate results. Foot Ankle Int 2005;26(10): 783–92.
34. Mann RA, Thompson FM. Arthrodesis of the first metatarsophalangeal joint for hallux valgus in rheumatoid arthritis. J Bone Joint Surg Am 1984;66(5):687–92.

Bunionette: Is There a Minimally Invasive Solution?

Frederick Michels, MD[a,b,c,*], Stéphane Guillo, MD[b,d]

KEYWORDS

- Bunionette • Tailor's bunion minimally invasive • Percutaneous
- Metatarsal osteotomy • Forefoot surgery • Fifth metatarsal

KEY POINTS

- The percutaneous technique is safe and reliable. The learning curve is small.
- The clinical and radiographic results are similar to conventional open procedures.
- The major advantage of the percutaneous technique is the limited risk of complications. This is due to the minimally invasive approach and the hardware-free technique.

INTRODUCTION

A bunionette deformity, or tailor's bunion, is a prominence of the fifth metatarsal head. The problem is similar to a bunion, except that a bunionette occurs on the outside of the foot. This lesion was described by Davies in 1949.[1] This deformity is 3 to 10 times more common in women than in men.[2] The most common symptoms are discomfort in certain shoes, pain, hyperkeratosis, and chronic ulcerations (**Fig. 1**).

Standard weight-bearing radiographs in 3 planes (lateral, anteroposterior, and oblique) are recommended if further assessment of the bone is needed. The following 2 angles are commonly used: the 4 to 5 intermetatarsal (IM) angle and the fifth metatarsophalangeal (MTP) angle (**Fig. 2**).

- The 4 to 5 IM angle is formed by the bisection of the line of the longitudinal axis of the fourth and fifth metatarsals. Divergence of the fourth and fifth metatarsals leads to pressure over the lateral eminence of the fifth metatarsal head. A 4 to 5 IM angle greater than 10° can be considered abnormal.[3]

There are no conflicts of interest with regard to this article.
[a] Orthopaedic Department, AZ Groeninge, President Kennedylaan 4, Kortrijk 8500, Belgium;
[b] Ankle Instability Group; [c] GRECMIP - MIFAS (Groupe de Recherche et d'Etude en Chirurgie Mini-Invasive du Pied - Minimally Invasive Foot and Ankle Society), Mérignac, France;
[d] Orthopaedic Department, Merignac Sport Clinic, 4, Rue Georges Negrevergne, Merignac 33700, France
* Corresponding author. Orthopaedic Department, AZ Groeninge, President Kennedylaan 4, Kortrijk 8500, Belgium.
E-mail address: frederick_michels@hotmail.com

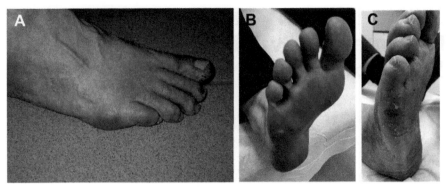

Fig. 1. Clinical aspect. (*A*) Painful prominence. (*B*) Hyperkeratosis. (*C*) Chronic ulcerations.

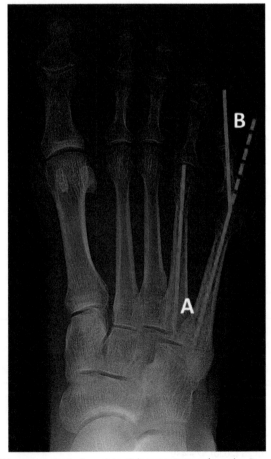

Fig. 2. Radiographic assessment. A = 4 to 5 intermetatarsal angle; B = angle of the fifth metatarsophalangeal joint.

- The angle of the fifth MTP joint measures the magnitude of medial deviation of the fifth toe in relation to the axis of the fifth metatarsal shaft. In most normal cases, the angle is 14° or less.[4]

In general, angular measurements serve only to describe a bunionette deformity. It is not the magnitude of the deformity that necessitates specific surgical treatment.

Classification

Du Vries distinguished 3 types according to the bony aspect.[5]

- Type 1 bunionette deformity: a prominent lateral condyle of the fifth metatarsal.
- Type 2 bunionette deformity: a lateral bowing of the diaphysis of the fifth metatarsal shaft.
- Type 3 bunionette deformity: a divergence of the fourth and fifth metatarsals. This is the most frequent type.

Associated Pathology

An associated deformity of the fifth toe is common. This can be a hammertoe, or supraductus or infraductus deformity. The bunionette is often seen in splayfoot disorders and many times accompanied with a hallux valgus.

INDICATIONS AND CONTRAINDICATIONS
Surgical Indications

In the first instance, nonoperative treatment is used to manage the symptoms. This includes shoe wear modification (a good, well-supported, wide toe box shoe), nonsteroidal anti-inflammatory medication, orthoses, and insoles.

Surgical treatment is performed when symptoms of an unacceptable degree are not relieved by conservative treatments.

Special Indications

- Congenital deformations can also lead to certain locations of hyper pressure. In particular, a congenital duplication of the fifth ray causes a larger foot with clinical signs of bunionette (**Fig. 3**). A percutaneous approach can be considered in those cases.
- Diabetic patients are at risk to develop recurrent ulcerations on the fifth metatarsal head (**Fig. 4**). These patients are the ideal indications to treat with a percutaneous technique to limit the risk to develop wound healing problems in the postoperative period.
- Patients with major vascular problems resulting in chronic wounds and exposed bone are relative contraindications for a percutaneous technique. As bone is probably infected, a partial resection metatarsal should be considered.

SURGICAL TECHNIQUE
History

The percutaneous technique was initially described by De Prado and colleagues[6] and Isham and colleagues.[7] The technique is based on the Reverdin-Isham procedure for the correction of hallux valgus.[7] In these first publications, several variations are described: condylectomy, distal osteotomy, middiaphyseal osteotomy, proximal osteotomy, and combined distal and proximal osteotomy.

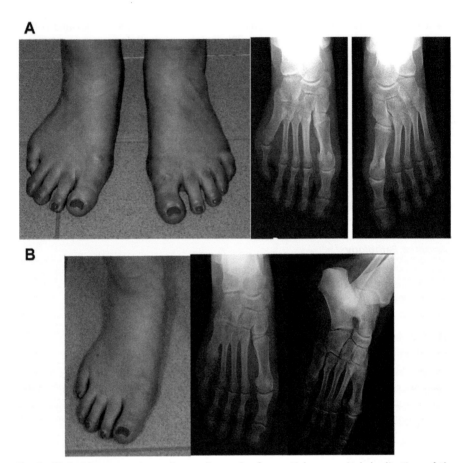

Fig. 3. Clinical image and standing radiograph of a partial congenital duplication of the fifth ray. (*A*) Preoperative images. (*B*) Images 3 months postoperatively.

Current Technique

Preparation and patient positioning

The patient is placed in supine position (**Fig. 5**). No tourniquet is used. The foot hangs over the edge of the operating table, with the contralateral limb bended. A mini C-arm is placed at the end of table. A micromotor with foot pedal is used.

First Step: Condylectomy

A condylectomy can be performed to resect bone on the lateral part of the metatarsal head. The earlier descriptions of the percutaneous technique routinely perform a condylectomy.[6,8,9] However, according to the more recent publications this step is rarely necessary.[10–12] As in open techniques, a condylectomy without osteotomy offers only limited correction. A condylectomy should not be performed if open growth plates are still present. However, in case of a bony spur a condylectomy is strongly recommended (**Fig. 6**). If both a condylectomy and osteotomy are performed, it is important to start with the condylectomy before the metatarsal osteotomy. In the inverse order the metatarsal head would be to unstable to perform the condylectomy.

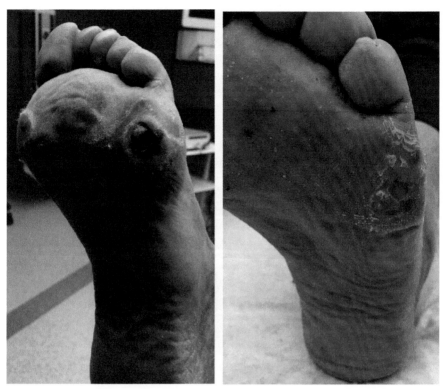

Fig. 4. Diabetic patient with chronic ulceration below the metatarsal head. Clinical image before surgery and after 3 months.

A Beaver Miniblade 64 is used to perform an incision on the plantar aspect just proximal of the metatarsal head (**Fig. 7**). The Beaver blade is used to detach the soft tissues from the bone and to create working space. The lateral hypertrophied aspect of the fifth metatarsal is removed with a long Shannon burr (2 × 12 mm). Using the burr, a glancing movement is performed to avoid irregularities. The resulting bone paste is removed by compression of the skin. The remaining fragments can be resected with a mini bone rasp. The bone resection is checked with a mini-C-arm fluoroscopy. Too much pressure on the burr can cause an irregular surface and irritation. Large fragments should be avoided because they are difficult to resect.

As in other percutaneous techniques, some precautions are needed to avoid burns. The velocity of the burr is limited to 7000 rounds per minute. During drilling, cooling with drips of water is important to prevent burning of the soft tissues. The burr should be cleaned regularly to retain the cutting capacities during the entire procedure.

Osteotomy

The osteotomy is the most commonly used technique. It can be partial or complete. A partial osteotomy allows les correction but faster bone healing.

The osteotomy can be performed at different locations. In case of an important widening of the 4 to 5 IM angle, a proximal osteotomy can be considered. However, this increases the risk of a delayed bone healing and other complication.[13] Some algorithms have been described but they are not commonly used in clinical studies.[14,15]

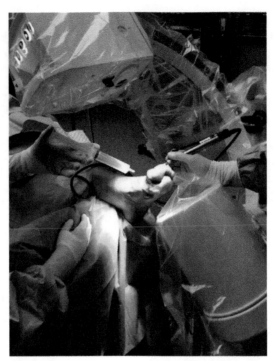

Fig. 5. Positioning with foot hanging over the edge of the table.

In our experience, most deformities can be corrected using 1 single osteotomy. In case of a bowing of the fifth metatarsal, the top of bowing is searched for by use of the fluoroscopy. In other types of deformity, the distal third of the diaphysis can be used. In general, a distal osteotomy is related to a lower risk of complications than a proximal osteotomy.[13]

A dorsal incision is made over the shaft of the fifth metatarsal, just next to the extensor tendon (**Fig. 8**). The soft tissues are dissected from the bone. Using a long Shannon burr (2 × 12 mm), an oblique osteotomy is performed from dorsal distal to plantar proximal (**Fig. 9**). An oblique osteotomy minimizes the risk to dorsal displacement and development of a transfer lesion beneath the fourth metatarsal head. When the osteotomy is completed, the distal part migrates medially. The different steps of the procedure are checked with the fluoroscopy (**Fig. 10**). External manual compression can be helpful to increase the correction.

Because of the very limited approach, wound closure is not necessary.

Additional Procedures

Some additional procedures are very often necessary because of an associated toe deformation.

Medial Capsulotomy

In case of an associated dorsal-adduction deformity of the fifth toe, a medial capsulotomy is needed. This can also be performed percutaneously. A small dorsal incision is performed on the medial side of the metatarsophalangeal joint. A mini Beaver blade

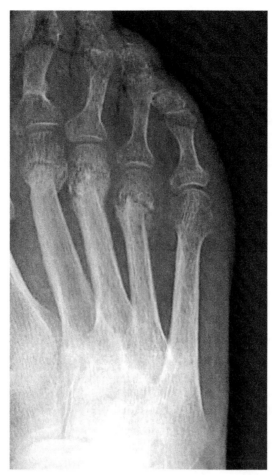

Fig. 6. Radiographic image of patient with sharp bone spur.

is introduced into the joint space with the sharp edge directed to the joint capsule and the collateral ligament. A valgus movement of the toe completes the capsulotomy.

Flexor Tenotomy

In case of a hammertoe deformity, a flexor tenotomy can be performed. The flexor tendon is incised on the middle of the proximal phalanx.

Phalangeal Osteotomy

Using the same plantar approach, a phalangeal osteotomy can be performed. This is needed in case of an important deviation of the proximal phalanx.

Extensor Tenotomy

In case of a supraductus toe deformity, an extensor tenotomy is performed. The extensor tendon is incised on the dorsal site of the metatarsophalangeal joint. Usually, a dorsal capsulotomy is associated.

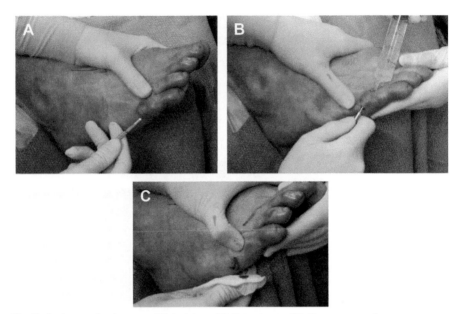

Fig. 7. Perioperative images. (*A*) Incision. (*B*) Osteotomy. (*C*). Bone removal.

POSTOPERATIVE MANAGEMENT

Postoperative dressings are extremely important. A splint dressing is applied to keep the intermetatarsal angle closed and the fifth toe in the right position. The first dressing change occurs 7 to 10 days postoperatively (**Fig. 11**). The splint dressing is used until 3 weeks postoperatively.

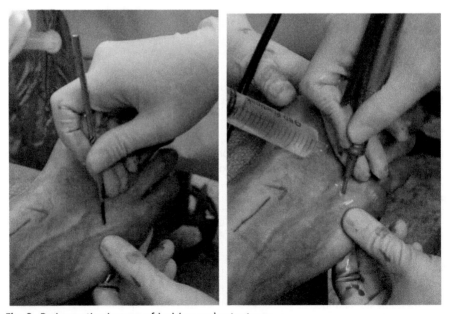

Fig. 8. Perioperative images of incision and osteotomy.

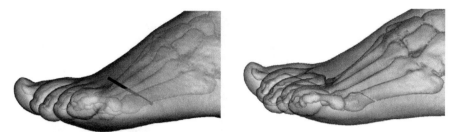

Fig. 9. Three-dimensional images of the osteotomy.

The patient is instructed to keep the foot in elevation for 1 week. This is important to limit pain, swelling, wound problems, and complex regional pain syndrome.

The patient is allowed to ambulate in a postoperative shoe for 4 to 6 weeks. In a next step, normal large shoes can be worn.

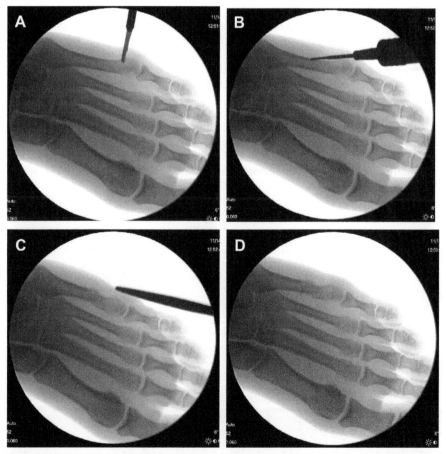

Fig. 10. Fluoroscopic images of the percutaneous metatarsal osteotomy. (*A*) Localization of the osteotomy site and incision. (*B*) Osteotomy with burr. (*C*) Translation by external pressure. (*D*) Final result.

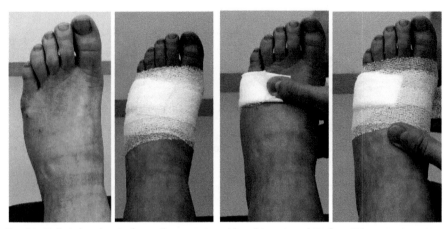

Fig. 11. Splint dressing to keep the metatarsal head in a translated position.

At 6 weeks, radiographs are taken (**Fig. 12**). Usually, first signs of callus formation can be seen. However, the stability of the osteotomy is assessed by clinical examination. A pain-free osteotomy site corresponds to a stable bone healing. The further activities should be adapted to the pain on the osteotomy site. Overuse should be avoided because this increases the risk to delayed bone union. In most cases the osteotomy is consolidated between 6 weeks and 3 months postoperatively (**Fig. 13**). Afterward, bone remodeling takes place.

A radiographic aspect of delayed bone healing is a well-known phenomenon after percutaneous surgery on the lateral metatarsals.[16] Clinical healing usually precedes radiographic evidence of bone healing by several weeks. This is a normal postoperative course and we should not be tempted to add some internal fixation.

Physiotherapy is only recommended if associated procedures (eg, hallux valgus correction, toe corrections) are performed.

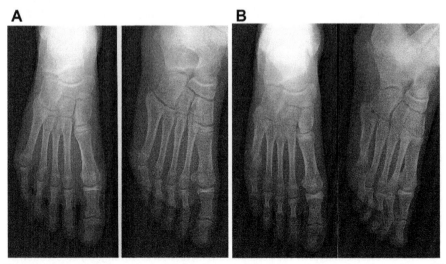

Fig. 12. Radiographs in patient with bunionette deformity and open growth cartilage. (*A*) Preoperative image. (*B*) Radiograph 6 weeks after osteotomy.

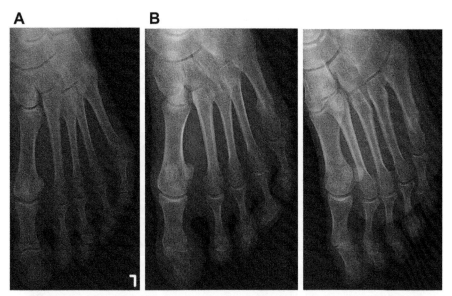

Fig. 13. Radiographs in patient with bunionette deformity and open growth cartilage. (*A*) Preoperative image. (*B*) Radiograph 3 months after osteotomy.

OUTCOME

A recent review study analyzed the results of 2 different minimally invasive techniques to treat bunionette deformity.[17] The first technique corresponded to the technique described in this article and 3 studies were included.[9,10,18] The second technique corresponded to a distal osteotomy of the fifth metatarsal combined with a percutaneously placed K-wire to keep the distal part in a translated position. Six studies using this technique were included.[19–24] The clinical results were assessed in all included studies. All studies reported good to excellent results. Postoperatively, mean American Orthopaedic Foot and Ankle Society (AOFAS) scores ranged from 88.2 to 100 points. In particular, the mean postoperative scores for techniques with and without fixation were 93.5 and 97.8, respectively. Patient satisfaction was high for both techniques. Correction of the 4 to 5 IM angle and the fifth MTP angle were similar in both groups.

Martijn and colleagues[13] performed a meta-analysis including 28 studies. All groups of osteotomies achieved significant 4 to 5 IM angle changes, with proximal osteotomies resulting in significantly greater changes than diaphyseal or distal osteotomies. All techniques demonstrated a significant improvement in the AOFAS scale scores compared with the preoperative situation. They reported an overall mean success rate of 93%.

COMPLICATIONS

The limited risk of complications is one of the main advantages of this percutaneous technique. This is for 2 reasons: the minimally invasive approach and the hardware-free technique.

- First, as in other minimally invasive techniques, the percutaneous approach limits the damage to the soft tissues. This avoids some complications, such as wound healing problems an infections. Especially in patients with an increased risk of wound healing problems, such as diabetic individuals and tobacco users, this

offers an important advantage. However, thermal injuries because of heating by the burrs can occur. They cause delayed wound healing and infection. As discussed previously, they can be avoided by using a careful surgical technique. Limitation of the speed and cooling of the burrs with saline irrigation is essential.
- Second, the hardware-free technique is also a major advantage. The recent meta-analysis of Martijn and colleagues[13] related more than one-half of the

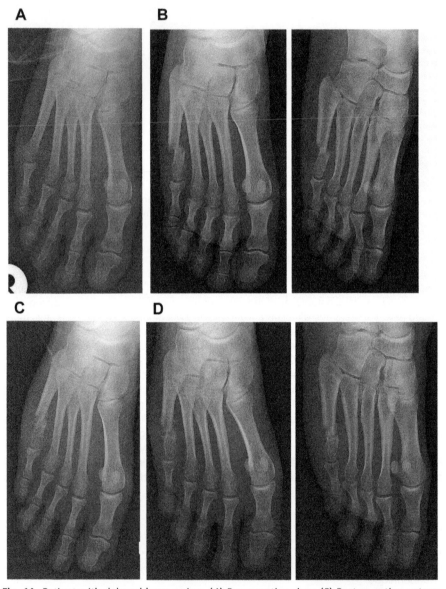

Fig. 14. Patient with delayed bone union. (*A*) Preoperative view. (*B*) Postoperative anteroposterior and oblique view. (*C*) Postoperative anteroposterior view after 6 weeks. (*D*) Postoperative anteroposterior and oblique view after 3 months: delayed bone healing. (*E*) Postoperative anteroposterior and oblique view after 6 months: hypertrophic callous. (*F*) Postoperative anteroposterior view after 2 years: bone remodeling.

E   F

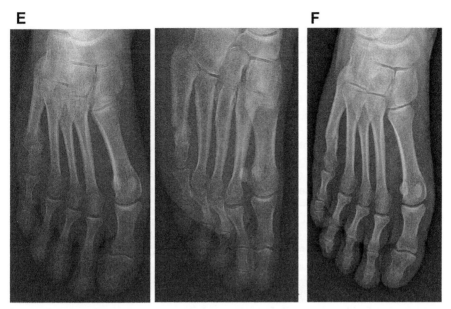

Fig. 14. (continued)

surgical complications to hardware. Screws can break and migrate. They can cause pain or irritation. Removal can be difficult.

The most encountered complication after a percutaneous bunionette correction is delayed union (**Fig. 14**).[9,10] A delayed union can develop when higher impact activities are restarted too early. At first this causes a delayed bone healing. Next a hypertrophic callus can develop, which can provoke occasional pain during several months. The callus and complaints usually disappear after 6 months.

Nerve lesions have not been reported in the clinical studies. A cadaveric study found no macroscopic nerve lesions after dissection of 20 specimens.[25] A recent cadaveric study used the clock method to locate the dorsolateral branch of the fifth toe.[26] This branch was found in all cases on the dorsolateral aspect of the fifth metatarsal. For this reason, a dorsomedial approach may decrease the risk to nerve lesions.

Vascular lesions have not been reported in clinical studies. The nutrient artery supplying the fifth metatarsal enters around the junction of the middle and proximal thirds of the medial aspect of the fifth metatarsal.[27] A damage of the vascular supply to the fifth metatarsal has been reported in open techniques performing proximal osteotomies.[28] This damage to the blood supply may explain a higher risk of complications, as nonunion and delayed union in more proximal osteotomies.

DIFFICULTY LEVEL AND LEARNING CURVE

As with all percutaneous techniques, it is vital that the surgeons engage in training on sawbones and cadaveric specimens before introducing them in clinical practice. However, the learning curve for bunionette surgery is small.[25] Fifth ray abnormalities have been described as the ideal indication for percutaneous surgery, given the simplicity of the procedure and postoperative course, high reliability, and very low rate of iatrogenic complications.[29]

REFERENCES

1. Davies H. Metatarsus quintus valgus. Br Med J 1949;1:664–5.
2. Roukis TS. The Tailor's bunionette deformity: a field guide to surgical correction. Clin Podiatr Med Surg 2005;22:223–45.
3. Coughlin MJ. Treatment of bunionette deformity with longitudinal diaphyseal osteotomy with distal soft tissue repair. Foot Ankle 1991;11:195–203.
4. Steel MW, Johnson KA, DeWitz MA, et al. Radiographic measurements of the normal adult foot. Foot Ankle 1980;1:151–8.
5. Du Vries HL. Surgery of the foot. 2nd edition. St Louis (MO): CV Mosby; 1965. p. 456–62.
6. De Prado M, Ripoll PL, Golano P. Cirugia percutanea del pie. Tecnicas quirurgicas, indicaciones, bases anatomicas. 1st edition. Barcelona (Spain): Masson Elsevier; 2003. p. p129–48.
7. Isham SA. The Reverdin-Isham procedure for the correction of hallux abducto valgus. A distal metatarsal osteotomy. Clin Podiatr Med Surg 1991;8:81–94.
8. Michels F, Guillo S, GRECMIP. Tailor's bunionectomy. In: Saxena A, editor. International advances in foot and ankle surgery. London: Springer; 2012. p. p99–106.
9. Michels F, Van Der Bauwhede J, Guillo S, et al. Percutaneous bunionette correction. Foot Ankle Surg 2013;19:9–14.
10. Laffenêtre O, Millet-Barbé B, Darcel V, et al. Percutaneous bunionette correction: results of a 49-case retrospective study at a mean 34 months' follow-up. Orthop Traumatol Surg Res 2015;101(2):179–84.
11. Molenaers B, Vanlommel J, Deprez P. Percutaneous hardware free corrective osteotomy for bunionnette deformity. Acta Orthop Belg 2017;83(2):284–91.
12. Teoh KH, Hariharan K. Minimally invasive distal metatarsal metaphyseal osteotomy (DMMO) of the fifth metatarsal for bunionette correction. Foot Ankle Int 2018;39(4):450–7.
13. Martijn HA, Sierevelt IN, Wassink S, et al. Fifth metatarsal osteotomies for treatment of bunionette deformity: a meta-analysis of angle correction and clinical condition. J Foot Ankle Surg 2018;57(1):140–8.
14. Morawe GA, Schmieschek MHT. Minimally invasive bunionette correction. Oper Orthop Traumatol 2018;30(3):184–94.
15. Redfern D, Vernois J, Legré BP. Percutaneous surgery of the forefoot. Clin Podiatr Med Surg 2015;32:291–332.
16. Bauer T, Laffenêtre O. Complications de la chirurgie percutanée de l'avant pied. In: Cazeau C, editor. Chirurgie mini-invasive et percutanée du pied. Montpellier (France): Sauramps Medical; 2009. p. 183–201.
17. Ceccarini P, Rinonapoli G, Nardi A, et al. Bunionette. minimally invasive and percutaneous techniques: a topical review of literature. Foot Ankle Spec 2017; 10(2):157–61.
18. Lui TH. Percutaneous osteotomy of the fifth metatarsal for symptomatic bunionette. J Foot Ankle Surg 2014;53(6):747–52.
19. Giannini S, Faldini C, Vannini F, et al. The minimally invasive osteotomy "SERI" (simple, effective, rapid, inexpensive) for correction of bunionette deformity. Foot Ankle Int 2008;29(3):282–6.
20. Legenstein R, Bonomo J, Huber W, et al. Correction of tailor's bunion with the Boesch technique: a retrospective study. Foot Ankle Int 2007;28:799–803.
21. Magnan B, Samaila E, Merlini M, et al. Percutaneous distal osteotomy of the fifth metatarsal for correction of bunionette. J Bone Joint Surg Am 2011;93:2116–22.

22. Martinelli R, Valentini R. Correction of valgus of fifth metatarsal and varus of the fifth toes by percutaneous distal osteotomy. Foot Ankle Surg 2007;13:136–9.
23. Waizy H, Olender G, Mansouri F, et al. Minimally invasive osteotomy for symptomatic bunionette deformity is not advisable for severe deformities: a critical retrospective analysis of the results. Foot Ankle Spec 2012;5:91–6.
24. Weitzel S, Trnka HJ, Petroutsas J. Transverse medial slide osteotomy for bunionette deformity: long-term results. Foot Ankle Int 2007;28:794–8.
25. Michels F, Guillo S, Cordier S, et al. A percutaneous bunionette correction: a cadaveric study. Clin Res Foot Ankle 2015;3:169.
26. Malagelada F, Dalmau-Pastor M, Sahirad C, et al. Anatomical considerations for minimally invasive osteotomy of the fifth metatarsal for bunionette correction - a pilot study. Foot (Edinb) 2018;36:39–42.
27. Tonogai I, Hayashi F, Tsuruo Y, et al. Direction and location of the nutrient artery to the fifth metatarsal at risk in osteotomy for bunionette. Foot Ankle Surg 2019; 25(2):193–7.
28. Diebold PF, Bejjani FJ. Basal osteotomy of the fifth metatarsal with intermetatarsal pinning: a new approach to tailor's bunion. Foot Ankle 1987;8:40–5.
29. Bauer T. Percutaneous forefoot surgery. Orthop Traumatol Surg Res 2014;100(1, suppl):S191–204.

Minimally Invasive Surgery: Osteotomies for Diabetic Foot Disease

Carlo Biz, MD[a,b,*], Pietro Ruggieri, MD, PhD[a]

KEYWORDS

- Minimally invasive surgery • Percutaneous surgery • Neuropathic ulcers
- Distal metatarsal osteotomies • Distal metatarsal diaphyseal osteotomies
- Metatarsalgia • Diabetic foot

KEY POINTS

- The treatment of diabetic foot ulcers is still challenging, but the application of minimally invasive surgery now represents a strategic management of these lesions to achieve health goals, highly uncertain until a few years ago.
- Minimally invasive distal metatarsal diaphyseal osteotomy (DMDO) is based on a distal osteotomy proximal to the metatarsal neck to reduce the pressure on the ulcer and favor its healing.
- The DMDO technique enables the restoration of the original harmonic distal parabola of the forefoot when possible, or the creation of a new balanced forefoot arch, promoting the healing of chronic pressure ulcers.
- This technique, in association with percutaneous osteotomies and tenotomies of phalanges, protects diabetic patients with minimal tissue damage, immediate postoperative weight bearing, and reduced risk of potential infections, because it does not require metal fixation.
- In a recent preliminary prospective study, DMDO was proved to be a safe and effective method for promoting the healing of chronic diabetic foot ulcers, regardless of their severity.

 Video content accompanies this article at http://www.foot.theclinics.com.

INTRODUCTION

The diabetic foot could seem hopeless because the prognosis of diabetic patients over the years often becomes inexorably worse. It is known that more than half of

[a] Department of Surgery, Oncology and Gastroenterology DiSCOG, Orthopedic and Traumatologic Clinic, University of Padova, Via Giustiniani 2, Padova 35128, Italy; [b] GRECMIP-MIFAS (Groupe de Recherche et d'Etude en Chirurgie Mini-Invasive du Pied-Minimally Invasive Foot and Ankle Society), Merignac, France
* Corresponding author. Department of Surgery, Oncology and Gastroenterology DiSCOG, Orthopedic and Traumatologic Clinic, University of Padova, Via Giustiniani 2, Padova 35128, Italy.
E-mail address: carlo.biz@unipd.it

Foot Ankle Clin N Am 25 (2020) 441–460
https://doi.org/10.1016/j.fcl.2020.05.006
1083-7515/20/© 2020 Elsevier Inc. All rights reserved.
foot.theclinics.com

all nontrauma amputations are done in diabetic patients because of a higher risk of developing peripheral vascular disease, deep infections, abscesses, osteomyelitis, or gangrene (**Fig. 1**) in an extremity.[1] In up to 84% cases,[2,3] the causative factor of these sequelae are diabetic foot ulcers (DFUs), the most common complication of diabetes type 1.[1] However, amputations may not be the most effective solution because they could be complicated by infections, which tend to be polymicrobial in diabetics (**Fig. 2**). Patients with pressure ulcers have a 2.5-fold increased risk of death compared with diabetic patients without DFUs. Further, DFU development is associated with 5% mortality during the first year and 42% mortality within 5 years.[4]

DFUs range from 2.2% in United Kingdom to 6.3% globally.[5] The prevalence of diabetic foot complication is lower for women than for men, and it is higher in patients affected by diabetes type 2 compared with those with diabetes type 1.[6] It is estimated that 19% to 34% of patients with diabetes are likely to be affected with a DFU during their lifetimes.[7] Because there is an increased number of newly diagnosed diabetics, the incidence of DFUs is expected to increase in the coming years.[8]

The cause of DFUs is multifactorial; peripheral neuropathy, poor glycemic control, calluses, foot deformities, improper foot care, ill-fitting footwear, peripheral artery disease, and dry skin are involved in the etiopathogenesis.[5,8] Their treatment continues to be challenging because of the high number of unhealed pressure ulcers found at 1 1year after treatment (20%) and because of the high recurrence rate of about 40% within 1 1year.[9]

At present, there is a new strategy: the successful application of minimally invasive surgery in the treatment of these dramatic lesions.[10] The distal metatarsal metaphyseal osteotomy (DMMO),[11] a technique used routinely in the last decade for the treatment of metatarsalgia, has been used to treat chronic plantar diabetic foot ulcers

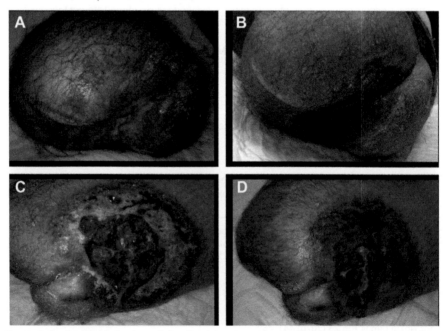

Fig. 1. Polymicrobial infection of the distal (*A, B*) and lateral (*C, D*) aspect of an above-knee amputation stump in a 48-year-old man.

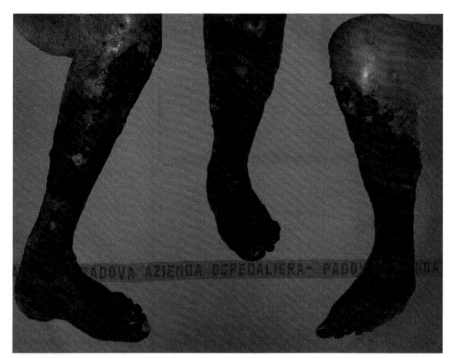

Fig. 2. Dry gangrene of the distal lower limb in a 52-year-old diabetic man with peripheral arterial disease and previous diabetic ulcers, who had refused amputation several times.

(CPDFUs).[12,13] A variant of this technique is the minimally invasive distal metatarsal diaphyseal osteotomy (DMDO).[13] This procedure is based on a distal osteotomy more proximal to the metatarsal neck, not only to reduce the pressure on the ulcer and consequently favoring its healing but also to restore the metatarsal parabola, preventing recurrent or transfer skin lesions.[13]

CLINICAL AND RADIOGRAPHIC APPROACH TO DIABETIC PATIENTS

There is substantial evidence from the literature that intensive foot care using a multidisciplinary approach is successful in reducing both hospitalization[14] and limb amputation rates in the diabetic population.[15–17] For this reason, in our center, it is routine practice for all patients with foot diabetic disease to be reviewed regularly by a multidisciplinary team. According to the institutional protocol, the clinical evaluation includes a complete clinical history of the patients, their characteristics (gender, age at the time of surgery, affected side, comorbidity, hemoglobin A1c, total CO_2, polymerase chain reaction, and peripheral vascular and neurologic status). The general aspects of the diabetic foot and related ulcers are evaluated. Routinely, the University of Texas Diabetic Wound Classification System[18,19] is used to grade CPDFUs (**Table 1**), whereas the ulcer's diameter and the major axes of the wounds are determined manually using a transparent sheet, as described by Coughlin and colleagues.[20]

In this way, patients with foot ulcers are evaluated for the most appropriate management: conservative or surgical. When the foot and ankle surgeon believes surgery is indicated, patients are referred for metatarsal percutaneous osteotomies and/or

Table 1
The University of Texas diabetic wound classification system

Ulcer	Grade			
Stage	0	I	II	III
A	Preulcerative or postulcerative lesion completely epithelialized	Superficial wound, not involving tendon, capsule, or bone	Wound penetrating to tendon or capsule	Wound penetrating to bone or joint
B	Preulcerative or postulcerative lesion completely epithelialized with infection	Superficial wound, not involving tendon, capsule, or bone with infection	Wound penetrating to tendon or capsule with infection	Wound penetrating to bone or joint with infection
C	Preulcerative or postulcerative lesion completely epithelialized with ischemia	Superficial wound, not involving tendon, capsule, or bone with ischemia	Wound penetrating to tendon or capsule with ischemia	Wound penetrating to bone or joint with ischemia
D	Preulcerative or postulcerative lesion completely epithelialized with infection and ischemia	Superficial wound, not involving tendon, capsule, or bone with infection and ischemia	Wound penetrating to tendon or capsule with infection and ischemia	Wound penetrating to bone or joint with infection and ischemia

Lavery LA, Armstrong DG, Harkless LB. Classification of diabetic foot wounds. J Foot Ankle Surg. 1996;35(6):528–31; with permission

lesser toe tenotomies. The number of metatarsal osteotomies that must be performed in each forefoot is planned according to how much the metatarsal formula is altered, following the Maestro criteria. In this way, it is decided where the osteotomies should lead to rebalance plantar pressures, to create a harmonious curve and to promote ulcer healing.[21] Further, in the cases of associated hallux valgus (HV) or claw toe deformities (CTDs), with or without ulcers, the local forefoot surgery protocol is followed. For HV, the surgery is Reverdin-Isham percutaneous osteotomy for mild to moderate HV deformity,[22] or the Endolog technique for moderate to severe HV deformity, both generally followed by percutaneous Akin osteotomy.[23] For toe deformities, the general treatment is as described by Redfern and Vernois,[24] recently simplified for diabetic patients with CTD.

SURGICAL TECHNIQUE
Surgical Procedures Described for Minimally Invasive Distal Metatarsal Diaphyseal Osteotomy Performed on the Left Foot by a Right-handed Surgeon (Videos)

- Patient position (Video 1): the patient must be in a supine position during the operation, with the operated foot protruding from the table. For 2 reasons, an ankle joint tourniquet is not required for this technique: blood is necessary to facilitate the removal of bone debris to be eliminated in the form of bone paste; and, more importantly, it is not indicated in diabetic lower limb surgery because of the problematic vascular peripheral system.

- Anesthesia: a regional block of the foot, involving deep nerves (deep peroneal and posterior tibial) and superficial nerves (saphenous, sural, and superficial peroneal) is recommended. A prophylactic antibiotic (cefazolin: 2 g) is administered before surgery.
- Equipment: a small scalpel blade (SM64), bone rasp, and periosteal elevator; a Shannon Isham burr (2.0 × 12 mm); a 20-mL syringe with normal saline solution; a fluoroscopy system for radiographic check; a power-driven burr, which has to provide a speed of approximately 2000 to 6000 rpm to avoid bone necrosis; bandages and tubular gauze for the final dressing.
- Portals (see Video 1): for surgery on a left foot by a right-handed surgeon, the top of the metatarsal head must first be palpated with the left thumb. Then, moving a few millimeters proximally at this level in the interspace on the right side of the head (ie, the lateral side for the left foot), an incision of 5 mm is made parallel to the extensor tendons by a small scalpel blade (SM64) at the dorsal side of the medial (or lateral) border of each metatarsal head that needs to be shortened. Care must be taken to avoid the network of veins at this level, which is usually visible because of the vasodilatation after the previous ankle block. The side of the incision depends on whether the surgeon is right or left handed; which foot is being operated on; and, more importantly, how much the metatarsal bone (MB) must be shortened in order to lift its head and facilitate the healing of the CPDFU.
- Osteotomy site (Video 2): the scalpel is moved forward at an oblique angle of about 45° until it reaches the dorsal aspect of the distal MB, proximal to the neck, to undergo osteotomy. Through the same incision, first a bone rasp specific for percutaneous surgery is inserted, and the periosteum is separated at the level of the osteotomy. A path is then prepared for the burr by using a periosteal elevator and positioning it obliquely at a 45° angle to the metatarsal axis, against the neck, which can be done by feel, using the instrument to move along the flare on the proximal part of the neck, from neck to distal diaphysis, mirroring the movement needed then for the osteotomy and detaching the tissues, which tend to be very stiff in diabetic feet.
- Osteotomy (Videos 3 and 4): a Shannon Isham burr (2.0 × 12 mm) is introduced until it reaches the metatarsal neck. It is then retracted a few millimeters proximally where the periosteum was previously removed. Fluoroscopy allows confirmation of the correct position of the osteotomy site on the distal diaphysis of the MB. In this position, cutting is started with an angle of approximately 45° with respect to the long axis of the MB in a dorsal-distal to proximal-plantar direction, with rotary motion, extending to the contralateral cortex (**Fig. 3**A). The lateral cortical surface is cut first in this way, then the plantar, medial, and lastly the dorsal cortical surface. Beginning with the section of the lateral cortex, the osteotomy is started with the motorized burr moving in a plantar and medial direction and ends with the section of the dorsal cortex, which is performed by pivoting in a rotational movement from the point of skin entry, involving a supination of the wrist of 90°. Thus, the burr comes to lie nearly flat on the foot at 90° to the metatarsal axis in the anteroposterior plane.
- Portal irrigation (see Video 4): the incision site is irrigated by normal saline during osteotomy because the burr can cause excessive heat, first burning the skin and subsequently resulting in fibrosis and pseudoarthrosis at the bone level.[22,25] The

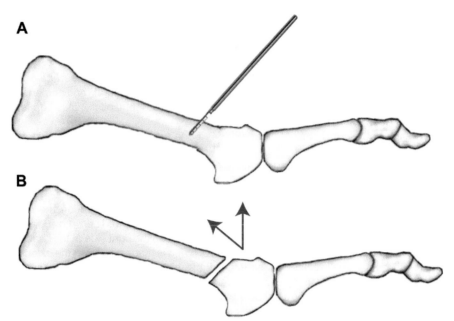

Fig. 3. The DMDO is performed with a 12-mm Shannon Isham burr with an angle of approximately 45° with respect to the long axis of the MB in a dorsal-distal to proximal-plantar direction (A). Hence, an ideal osteotomy has been performed proximal to the neck with potentially greater elevation of metatarsal head from the ground (B).

lavage is also useful to remove bone debris, preventing periarticular ossifications in the stab canal.

- Compacting of osteotomy sides (Video 5): the bone is manually compacted on completion of the osteotomy by exercising pressure in the distal-proximal direction of the MB of interest, pushing the metatarsal head dorsally and producing contact of the trabecular bone, because no internal fixation is performed. The toe must be mobilized along the metatarsal axis to ensure that the metatarsal heads can move together under full weight bearing. This movement allows mobilization of periosteal adhesions that could promote the shortening and elevation of the distal part of the MB during walking (**Fig. 3**B).
- Ulcer debridement: by accurate ulcer debridement, the CPDFU is converted into an acute wound in order to enable the normal stages of healing,[26,27] whereas resorbable sutures should be used to close the rest of the wounds.

Tenotomies and Osteotomies for Lesser Toe Deformities

As stated by Redfern and Vernois,[24] percutaneous surgical techniques are particularly effective for the correction of lesser toe deformities and may be advantageous in cases considered at higher risk of cutaneous or vascular complications, such as diabetes and neuropathic feet. Hence, ulcers at the dorsal aspect of the proximal interphalangeal (PIP) joint, usually caused by rubbing against the toe box of shoes, can be prevented in areas of hyperkeratosis or treated through multiple percutaneous tenotomies and phalangeal osteotomies of the lesser toes.

For these different procedures, anesthesia and antibiotic prophylaxis, patient position without tourniquet, minimally invasive equipment, and portal irrigation are the same as in DMDO, except for the burr, which should be a Shannon Isham burr (2.0 × 8 mm).

In our experience, to simplify this surgery, we apply Piclet's technique as originally described in 2009[28] and published in 2018:[29]

- Tenotomies (Video 6): by a short plantar incision just proximal to the metatarsophalangeal joint (MTPJ), a flexor digitorum brevis tenotomy, followed by a second plantar incision at the level of PIP for its release, and flexor digitorum longus (FDL) tenotomy are performed in patients with flexible deformity.
- Phalanx osteotomies (Video 7): through the first plantar incision, associated P1, and sometimes P2, osteotomies are also performed in patients with fixed deformity.
- Toe extension (see Video 7): finally, to obtain proper correction in both cases, a forced extension is always applied as well as a final extensor digitorum longus/extensor digitorum brevis tenotomy only when further improvement of the correction is required.

Bandage

The bandage is very important to maintain the correction obtained after surgery because there is no osteosynthesis material in this operation. Surgeons wishing to attempt these techniques must be familiar with the proper wrapping of the bandage to control the metatarsal axis and toe position in the postoperative period while healing occurs.

- Tape is used for bandages, which are bent and crisscrossed, tracing between all intermetatarsal spaces, crossing them over the medial (lateral) aspect of each of the osteotomies performed (depending on the foot side) to reinforce the strength of the bandage.
- To maintain the toe in slight plantar inclination, gentle traction is used.
- Tubular gauze is used to cover the forefoot, except for the distal part of the toes and nails to check distal vascularization of the foot.

Postoperative Care

According to our postoperative protocol:
- Before the patient's discharge, anteroposterior and lateral radiographs of non–weight-bearing feet should be taken.
- The day after surgery, the patients are allowed to walk using a rigid flat-soled orthopedic shoe for the following 30-day period. (This is very important because metatarsal length is set automatically on weight bearing of the foot.[22])
- Oral antibiotic prophylaxis for a week is recommended starting from the day of the surgery, as well as thromboembolic prophylaxis (natrium enoxaparin: 4000 IU/d) and an antiedemigen therapy (Leucoselect, Lymphaselect, and Bromelina: 1 tablet/day) for 30 days. An analgesic therapy is prescribed for 2 weeks (etoricoxib, 60 mg, 1 tablet/day in the morning), also to prevent heterotopic ossification when comorbidities of the patient permit it, or alternatively, paracetamol (1 g, 1 tablet x2/day).
- Each of the patients is seen once a week for a month on an outpatient basis. The first control is 8 days after surgery. The original bandage is removed and substituted by a simpler bandage. At the next 3 weekly visits, the bandage is changed in the same way.
- The bandage is totally removed 1 month after surgery if the ulcer is completely closed, and anteroposterior weight-bearing and lateral radiographs are taken. The patient is then able to walk with comfortable shoes or orthopedic footwear

(according to previous foot deformity), allowing total load on the operated foot. If the ulcer is not completely healed, the patient is seen every week for medication until total healing of the lesion.

Indications and Contraindications

Percutaneous procedures correcting foot deformities, thereby decreasing plantar pressure by internal floating metatarsal and phalangeal osteotomies in case of rubbing against the toe box of shoes, are indicated when conservative methods fail, usually after at least 6 weeks of off-loading orthotic treatment and standard conservative treatment. The general indications are largely the same as for metatarsal head resection, arthroplasty resection, and bunionette correction.[30,31] Further, because of the tiny percutaneous portal incisions, the osteotomies and tenotomies of the forefoot can often be considered in situations where there is poor local soft tissue, or previous amputations of toes and/or MBs with scarring. During the operation, the number of metatarsal osteotomies performed in each forefoot is planned according to how much the metatarsal formula of preoperative radiographs was altered according to the Maestro criteria.[12,13,21] It should generally be considered almost obligatory to perform the osteotomies to the second, third, and fourth MBs in order to avoid a transfer lesion developing under the third or fourth metatarsal heads. The presence of significant arthritis and stiffness in the associated MTPJ and the consequent association of reported increased risk of nonunion in this situation[12,24] is not a contraindication for DMDO, as it is a diaphyseal osteotomy. In addition, the authors strongly believe that ulcers with chronic infection, or ulcers penetrating deep structures (IIIB), osteomyelitis of the MBs or the distal phalanx, ankle brachial index less than 0.5, or flat pulse volume recording at the ankle level are relative, but not absolute, contraindications for the procedure in the absence of associated cellulitis.

On the contrary, the few absolute contraindications of these percutaneous procedures are:

- Severe ischemia and gangrene
- Insufficient vascular perfusion
- Extensive soft tissue infection presenting as cellulitis of the foot or toe

Complications

The potential complications of these percutaneous techniques, mostly minor, have been well described[13,24,30,32,33]: ulcer recurrence, ulcer transfer, superficial infection, malunion, and nonunion. However, they are reported in lower percentages than those that occurred after standard care. In particular, persistent moderate swelling of the forefoot for more than 6 weeks without infection has been described, which has been resolved after complete callus formation at the osteotomy levels,[13] whereas, more recently, some cases of exuberant callus formation were noted.

To the best of our knowledge, no cases of major complications (deep wound infection, MB osteomyelitis or avascular necrosis of metatarsal head, and acute Charcot osteoarthropathy) have been reported in the literature. However, it is possible that, with longer follow-up (FU) and a larger patient group, an increase in the number of complications of this evolving disease could occur.

RESULTS

All these procedures were managed as described in the following case series.

Case 1

A 52-year-old female patient with a past medical history of type I diabetes, resolved after kidney and pancreas transplant. She presented with right foot distal neuropathy, HV, metatarsalgia, hyperkeratosis, fixed CTDs, having undergone DMDO of the second, third, and fourth metatarsal bone for a IIIB chronic ulcer extending into the MTPJ. Three years prior she had presented with a IIIB CPDFU over the lateral aspect of the MTPJ of the fifth ray of the same foot, caused by osteomyelitis. A transmetatar-sal amputation of the right foot was suggested at another institution, which the patient refused. She attended our orthopedic clinic for a second opinion, where a fifth MB head resection and minimally invasive regularization through the same ulcer was proposed with success. Clinical (**Fig. 4**) images at preoperative, 3-month, 6-month, and 72-month FU showed complete healing of both CPDFUs, reduction of the hyperkera-totic areas, and maintenance of the results obtained. Radiographic (**Fig. 5**) images at preoperative, 3-month, 6-month, and 72-month FU showed bone union and remodeling.

Case 2

A 68-year-old type II diabetic female patient having undergone percutaneous osteotomy of P1 of the second, third, and fourth toes, associated with percuta-neous FBB, FDL tenotomies, and PIP release for CTD of her right foot and percutaneous lengthening of hallux flexor tendon of her HV for recalcitrant IC ulcers of the toes. Clinical images (**Fig. 6**) at preoperative, 2-month, and 60-month FU showed complete healing of the ulcer and toe realignment without recurrence.

Case 3

A 67-year-old type II diabetic male patient having undergone DMDO of the fourth and fifth MBs for a IB CPDFU. Clinical (**Fig. 7**) and radiographic (**Fig. 8**) images at preop-erative, 1-month, 3-month, and 52-month FU showed complete healing of the ulcer and bone union.

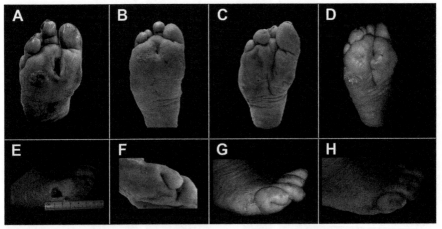

Fig. 4. Case 1: clinical images at (*A-E*) preoperative, (*B-F*) 3-month, (*C-G*) 6-month, and (*D-H*) 72-month follow-up.

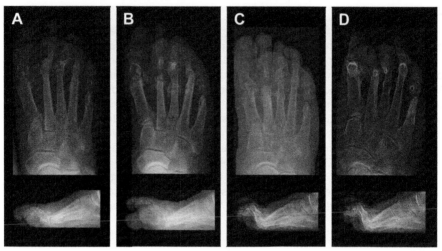

Fig. 5. Case 1: Radiographic images at (*A*) preoperative, (*B*) 3-month, (*C*) 6-month, and (*D*) 72-month follow-up.

Case 4

A 61-year-old type I diabetic male patient who underwent an Endolog technique for moderate-severe HV correction, percutaneous Akin osteotomy, DMDO of the second, third, fourth, and fifth MBs for a IIB CPDFU, percutaneous osteotomy of P1 of the second toe for associated fixed CTD and percutaneous FBB, FDL tenotomies, and PIP release of the second, third, fourth, and fifth toes for fixed (second) and flexible CTDs of his right foot. Clinical (**Fig. 9**) images at preoperative, 2-month, and 34-month

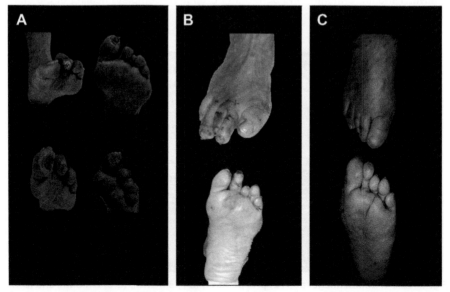

Fig. 6. Case 2: clinical images at (*A*) preoperative, (*B*) 2-month, and (*C*) 60-month follow-up.

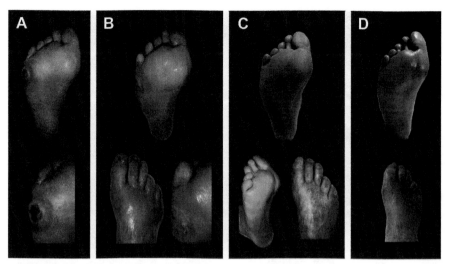

Fig. 7. Case 3: clinical images at (A) preoperative, (B) 1-month, (C) 3-month, and (D) 52-month follow-up.

FU and radiographic (**Fig. 10**) images at preoperative, 2-month, 6-month, and 34-month FU, showing complete healing of the ulcer and toe realignment, bone union with exuberant callus formation, and metatarsal rebalance.

Case 5

An 80-year-old type II diabetic male patient who had previously undergone bilateral forefoot amputations at another institution a few years prior came to our orthopedic clinic for recalcitrant IIIB CPDFUs on both feet. The proposed plan included a double DMDO of the third MB and a simple DMDO of the fourth and fifth MBs associated with percutaneous FBB, FDL tenotomies, and PIP release for flexible CTDs of

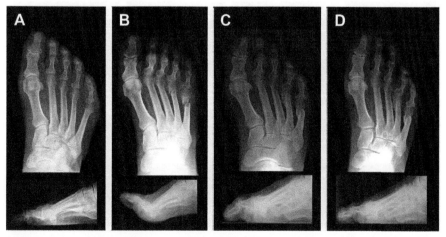

Fig. 8. Case 3: radiographic images at (A) preoperative, (B) 1-month, (C) 3-month, and (D) 52-month follow-up.

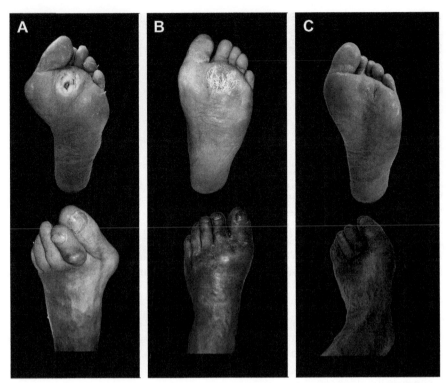

Fig. 9. Case 4: clinical images at (A) preoperative, (B) 2-month, and (C) 34-month follow-up.

the right foot. Clinical (**Fig. 11**) images at preoperative, 2-month, 3-month, and 6-month FU showed complete healing of the ulcer on the right foot; radiographic (**Fig. 12**) images at preoperative, 2-month, and 6-month FU showed bone union and remodeling.

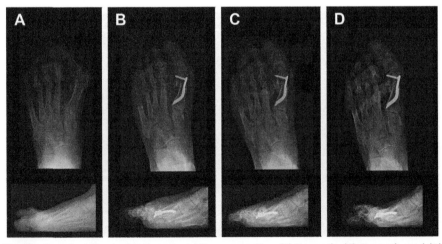

Fig. 10. Case 4: radiographic images at (A) preoperative, (B) 2-month, (C) 6-month, and (D) 34-month follow-up.

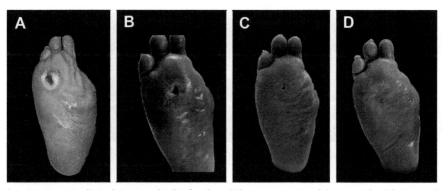

Fig. 11. Case 5: clinical images (right foot) at (*A*) preoperative, (*B*) 2-month, (*C*) 3-month, and (*D*) 6-month follow-up.

During the same operation, this patient underwent DMDO of the second and third MBs, associated with percutaneous FBB, FDL tenotomies, and PIP release for CTDs of the left foot. During the first month of weekly medications, the second metatarsal head had to be removed because of exposure through the ulcer. Clinical (**Fig. 13**) images at preoperative, 2-month, 3-month, and 6-month FU showed complete healing of the ulcer on the left foot. Radiographic (**Fig. 14**) images at preoperative, 2-month, and 6-month FU showed bone union and remodeling.

Case 6

As shown in the video clip, this 76-year-old type I diabetic man had undergone DMDO of the second, third, fourth, and fifth MBs for a IIB CPDFU, and percutaneous

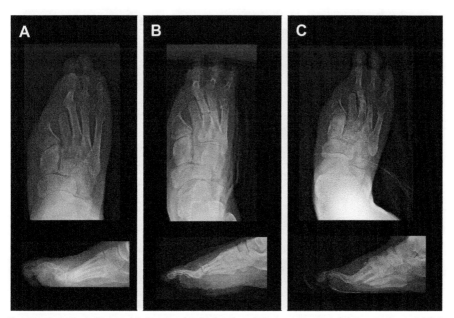

Fig. 12. Case 5: radiographic images (right foot) at (*A*) preoperative, (*B*) 2-month, and (*C*) 6-month follow-up.

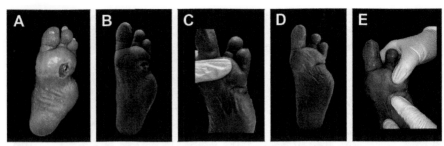

Fig. 13. Case 5: clinical images (left foot) at (*A*) preoperative, (*B*) 2-month, (*C*) 3-month, and (*E*) 6-month follow-up.

osteotomy of P1 of all lesser toes associated with percutaneous tenotomies and PIP release for CTDs of his right foot. Clinical images (**Fig. 15**) at preoperative, 1-month, 2-month, and 6-month FU showed the complete healing of both ulcers. Radiographic images are also provided (**Fig. 16**) at preoperative and 2-month FU. This case was complicated by a lengthy period of forced bed rest immediately after surgery for cardiology problems, therefore standing radiographs were not obtained during the following clinical FUs. Nonetheless, on the lateral radiograph projection, as marked by the red arrow, the metatarsal heads appear lifted (see **Fig. 16**B).

WHY SHOULD PERCUTANEOUS OSTEOTOMIES BE PERFORMED IN DIABETIC FOREFEET?
State of the Art

Within the last decade, the well-known DMMO and the innovative distal oblique metatarsal minimal invasive osteotomy (DOMMO) have proved to be alternative surgical

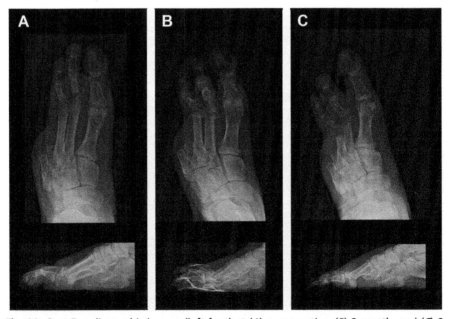

Fig. 14. Case 5: radiographic images (left foot) at (*A*) preoperative, (*B*) 2-month, and (*C*) 6-month follow-up.

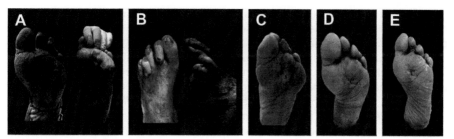

Fig. 15. Case 6: clinical images at (*A-B*) preoperative, (*C*) 1-month, (*D*) 2-month, and (*E*) 6-month follow-up.

approaches for central primary metatarsalgia.[11,24,34,35] More recently, this percutaneous procedure was modified to reduce the plantar pressure of the MBs over CPDFUs in diabetic patients, promoting ulcer healing.[13] In the 1990s, Vitti and colleagues[36] showed that the presence of diabetes is an independent predictor of poor healing after forefoot surgery, but many studies have found that the diabetic status fails to predict outcomes from limited amputation.[37,38] In this regard, the authors believe that any external insult to the diabetic foot could only worsen the diabetic status, leading to more proximal, and sometimes not even resolutive, amputation. For these reasons, percutaneous surgery is a valid alternative to traditional conservative treatments,[39] such as non–weight bearing for a long period and total contact

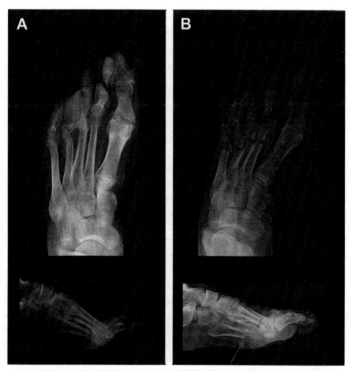

Fig. 16. Case 6: radiographic images at (*A*) preoperative and (*B*) 2-month follow-up, where the metatarsal heads appear lifted, as marked by the red arrow.

cast.[40–42] Afterward, continued care is required with special shoes and orthotics to prevent recurrence. Hence, these conservative methods often fail because of complications or lack of compliance.[43]

By its nature, minimally invasive surgery minimizes the tissue damage derived from surgical aggression, solving at the same time the mechanical causes that led to ulcer formation. The main purpose of this procedure is to decrease the pressure plantar to the affected metatarsal head. Further, because full weight bearing in a postoperative flat shoe is allowed immediately after surgery, the postoperative period is more comfortable for the patients. This result can also be achieved by more popular surgical techniques: plantar condylectomy, Weil osteotomy, closing wedge metatarsal osteotomy with metal fixation, and Helal osteotomy.[33,44–47] However, they tend to have high complication rates because of wound dehiscence and/or postoperative infections.

CPDFUs were initially hypothesized to be lesions caused by overactivity of both the long extensor and long flexor.[48] However, the authors believe that the major causative factor is not muscle imbalance but the progressive collapse of the transversal axis of the foot.[13] Because internal fixation is not used in the DMDO technique, avoiding potential infection of the metalwork, the osteotomized metatarsal heads are shifted, adapting to the load toward a new position, which is translated in a slightly dorsal direction, where the heads ossify. In this way, the use of percutaneous techniques enables:

- First, obtaining a better distribution of plantar pressure on the MBs, resulting in a lengthening of the load under the ulcer, promoting its rapid healing.[49,50]
- Second, restoring the original harmonic distal parabola of the forefoot when possible, or creating a new balanced forefoot arch. In order to respect the Maestro criteria,[21] it is often necessary to shorten the MB to a greater degree, performing a diaphyseal osteotomy much more proximal to the neck.

From the mechanical point of view, Redfern and Vernois[24] correctly stated that making the osteotomy more proximal to the neck is a technique error when performing DMMO, causing MB displacement in dorsal rotation and a consequent overelevation of the metatarsal head, making a DOMMO preferable in these cases. In contrast, this is exactly the main goal of performing DMDO for CPDFU treatment.

The applications of minimally invasive surgery for the treatment of diabetic disease is not new. In 1990, Tillo and colleagues[33] was the first to propose a dorsal osteoclasis at the level of the metatarsal neck for the treatment of DFUs, reporting a recurrence rate of 6% and a transfer lesion rate of 26.5% during a 17-month FU. In 1999, Fleischli and colleagues[32] described a dorsiflexion metatarsal base osteotomy fixed by pins for the treatment of CPDFU. Although good results were reported with a high healing rate (95%), complications occurred in 68% of cases, including acute Charcot disease, deep wound infections, and transfer ulcers.

A recent meta-analysis of the contemporary management of diabetic neuropathic foot ulcerations reveals disappointing functional outcomes,[31] and percutaneous surgery for CPDFUs by metatarsal osteotomies was found to be a poorly investigated topic. Contrary to the traditional surgical techniques, only 4 case series studies could be located in the literature.[31] In these analyses, despite the common association between decreased healing rates and severity and duration of CPDFUs,[31] the healing rates and time found by the different investigators proved far better than those reported with standard care in terms of ulcer duration and severity, knowing that included ulcers were all either recurrent or recalcitrant to initial standard care. Further, complications (ulcer recurrence, ulcer transfer, infection, and nonunion) were less frequent with respect to those reported following standard care.

Another recent evidence-based review challenges the classic guidelines on diabetic forefoot ulcer management.[31] It shows that off-loading surgery probably yields better outcomes than conservative treatment. Specifically, metatarsal head resection, arthroplasty resection, and metatarsal osteotomies at different levels generated excellent healing rates with short healing durations and low recurrence rates. Thus, these investigators concluded that floating osteotomies could be used more often and proposed earlier in the course of DFUs.

In the last few years, Tamir and colleagues[48] described the use of percutaneous tenotomies for the treatment of diabetic toe ulcers and mini-invasive floating osteotomies for the treatment of resistant or recurrent DFUs, reporting excellent results. Although they treated ulcers exclusively of University of Texas grade IA, their findings were confirmed by our results reported recently and updated in this article (42.9% of CPDFUs of grade IIIB).[13]

SUMMARY

The DMDO is an effective procedure for the treatment of complicated CPDFUs under the heads of lateral MBs (even the fifth), resistant toe ulcers, and recurrent pressure ulcers, mainly those with healing delay or as a consequence of previous forefoot amputations with unbalancing of the metatarsal formula. DMDO is effective even when associated with percutaneous extensor and flexor tenotomies in cases of CTD and percutaneous osteotomies of phalanges in case of fixed deformities. For diabetic patients, the main advantages of this method, performed by distal ankle block, without tourniquet, and with a very low risk of complications, are:

- Minimal surgical scars and tissue damage
- Immediately postoperative weight bearing
- Absence of osteosynthesis and consequent potential infection of metal fixation
- Reduction of the previous high plantar pressures by the restoration of a harmonic balanced forefoot arch
- Rapid ulcer healing

DISCLOSURE

The authors have nothing to disclose.

SUPPLEMENTARY DATA

Supplementary data related to this article can be found online at https://doi.org/10.1016/j.fcl.2020.05.006.

REFERENCES

1. Muduli IC, P P A, Panda C, et al. Diabetic foot ulcer complications and its management-a medical college-based descriptive study in odisha, an eastern state of India. Indian J Surg 2015;77(Suppl 2):270–4.

2. Prevention C. National diabetes statistics report: estimates of diabetes and its burden in the United States, 2014. Atlanta (GA): US Department of Health and Human Services; 2014.

3. Reiber GE. The epidemiology of diabetic foot problems. Diabet Med 1996;13(S1):S6–11.

4. Walsh JW, Hoffstad OJ, Sullivan MO, et al. Association of diabetic foot ulcer and death in a population-based cohort from the United Kingdom. Diabet Med 2016; 33(11):1493–8.

5. Armstrong DG, Boulton AJM, Bus SA. Diabetic foot ulcers and their recurrence. N Engl J Med 2017;376(24):2367–75.

6. International Diabetes Federation. IDF diabetes Atlas. 8th ed, Brussels 2017. Available at: http://www.diabetesatlas.org. Accessed November 16, 2019.

7. Singh N, Armstrong DG, Lipsky BA. Preventing foot ulcers in patients with diabetes. JAMA 2005;293(2):217–28.

8. Oliver TI, Mutluoglu M. Diabetic foot ulcer. In: StatPearls. Treasure Island (FL): StatPearls Publishing StatPearls Publishing LLC; 2019.

9. Everett E, Mathioudakis N. Update on management of diabetic foot ulcers. Ann N Y Acad Sci 2018;1411(1):153–65.

10. Batista F, Magalhaes AA, Nery C, et al. Minimally invasive surgery for diabetic plantar foot ulcerations. Diabet Foot Ankle 2011;2(1):10358.

11. Laffenêtre O, Perera A. Distal minimally invasive metatarsal osteotomy ("DMMO" Procedure). Foot Ankle Clin 2019;24(4):615–25.

12. Biz C, Corradin M, Kuete Kanah WT, et al. Medium-long-term clinical and radiographic outcomes of minimally invasive distal metatarsal metaphyseal osteotomy (DMMO) for central primary metatarsalgia: do maestro criteria have a predictive value in the preoperative planning for this percutaneous technique? Biomed Research International 2018;2018:1947024.

13. Biz C, Gastaldo S, Dalmau-Pastor M, et al. Minimally invasive distal metatarsal diaphyseal osteotomy (DMDO) for chronic plantar diabetic foot ulcers. Foot Ankle Int 2018;39(1):83–92.

14. Lavery LA, Wunderlich RP, Tredwell JL. Disease management for the diabetic foot: effectiveness of a diabetic foot prevention program to reduce amputations and hospitalizations. Diabetes Res Clin Pract 2005;70(1):31–7.

15. Al-Wahbi AM. Impact of a diabetic foot care education program on lower limb amputation rate. Vasc Health Risk Manag 2010;6:923–34.

16. Apelqvist J, Larsson J. What is the most effective way to reduce incidence of amputation in the diabetic foot? Diabetes Metab Res Rev 2000;16(Suppl 1): S75–83.

17. Van Gils CC, Wheeler LA, Mellstrom M, et al. Amputation prevention by vascular surgery and podiatry collaboration in high-risk diabetic and nondiabetic patients. The Operation Desert Foot experience. Diabetes Care 1999;22(5):678–83.

18. Lavery LA, Armstrong DG, Harkless LB. Classification of diabetic foot wounds. J Foot Ankle Surg 1996;35(6):528–31.

19. Oyibo SO, Jude EB, Tarawneh I, et al. A comparison of two diabetic foot ulcer classification systems: the Wagner and the University of Texas wound classification systems. Diabetes Care 2001;24(1):84–8.

20. Coughlin M, Mann R, Saltzman C. Surgery of the foot and ankle. Philadelphia: Mosby; 2007. p. 1289.

21. Maestro M, Besse J-L, Ragusa M, et al. Forefoot morphotype study and planning method for forefoot osteotomy. Foot Ankle Clin 2003;8(4):695–710.

22. Biz C, Fosser M, Dalmau-Pastor M, et al. Functional and radiographic outcomes of hallux valgus correction by mini-invasive surgery with Reverdin-Isham and Akin percutaneous osteotomies: a longitudinal prospective study with a 48-month follow-up. J Orthop Surg Res 2016;11(1):157.

23. Biz C, Corradin M, Petretta I, et al. Endolog technique for correction of hallux valgus: a prospective study of 30 patients with 4-year follow-up. J Orthop Surg Res 2015;10:102.

24. Redfern DJ, Vernois J. Percutaneous Surgery for Metatarsalgia and the Lesser Toes. Foot Ankle Clin 2016;21(3):527–50.

25. Muñoz-García N, Tomé-Bermejo F, Herrera-Molpeceres J. Pseudoarthrosis after distal percutaneous osteotomy of lower distal radii. Revista Española de Cirugía Ortopédica y Traumatología (English Edition) 2011;55(1):31–4.

26. Kim PJ, Steinberg JS. Wound care: biofilm and its impact on the latest treatment modalities for ulcerations of the diabetic foot. Semin Vasc Surg 2012;25(2):70–4.

27. Lebrun E, Tomic-Canic M, Kirsner RS. The role of surgical debridement in healing of diabetic foot ulcers. Wound Repair Regen 2010;18(5):433–8.

28. Piclet-Legre B. Traitement chirurgical percutané des déformations des orteils latéraux. In: Cazeau C, editor. Chirurgie mini-invasive et percutanée du pied, Sauramps Médical, Paris. 2009. p. 157–67.

29. Frey-Ollivier S, Catena F, Hélix-Giordanino M, et al. Treatment of flexible lesser toe deformities. Foot Ankle Clin 2018;23(1):69–90.

30. Tamir E, Finestone AS, Avisar E, et al. Mini-Invasive floating metatarsal osteotomy for resistant or recurrent neuropathic plantar metatarsal head ulcers. J Orthop Surg Res 2016;11(1):78.

31. Yammine K, Assi C. Surgical offloading techniques should be used more often and earlier in treating forefoot diabetic ulcers: an evidence-based review. Int J Low Extrem Wounds 2019. https://doi.org/10.1177/1534734619888361. 1534734619888361.

32. Fleischli JE, Anderson RB, Davis WH. Dorsiflexion metatarsal osteotomy for treatment of recalcitrant diabetic neuropathic ulcers. Foot Ankle Int 1999;20(2):80–5.

33. Tillo TH, Giurini JM, Habershaw GM, et al. Review of metatarsal osteotomies for the treatment of neuropathic ulcerations. J Am Podiatr Med Assoc 1990;80(4): 211–7.

34. De Prado M, Cuervas-Mons M, Golanó P, et al. Distal metatarsal minimal invasive osteotomy (DMMO) for the treatment of metatarsalgia. Tech Foot Ankle Surg 2016;15(1):12–8.

35. Khurana A, Kadamabande S, James S, et al. Assessment of medium term results and predictive factors in recurrent metatarsalgia. Foot Ankle Surg 2011;17(3): 150–7.

36. Vitti MJ, Robinson DV, Hauer-Jensen M, et al. Wound healing in forefoot amputations: the predictive value of toe pressure. Ann Vasc Surg 1994;8(1):99–106.

37. Byrne RL, Nicholson ML, Woolford TJ, et al. Factors influencing the healing of distal amputations performed for lower limb ischaemia. Br J Surg 1992; 79(1):73–5.

38. Yeager RA, Moneta GL, Edwards JM, et al. Predictors of outcome of forefoot surgery for ulceration and gangrene. Am J Surg 1998;175(5):388–90.

39. Finestone AS, Tamir E, Ron G, et al. Surgical offloading procedures for diabetic foot ulcers compared to best non-surgical treatment: a study protocol for a randomized controlled trial. J Foot Ankle Res 2018;11:6.

40. Bus SA, van Deursen RW, Armstrong DG, et al. Footwear and offloading interventions to prevent and heal foot ulcers and reduce plantar pressure in patients with diabetes: a systematic review. Diabetes Metab Res Rev 2016;32(Suppl 1): 99–118.

41. Bus SA, van Netten JJ, Lavery LA, et al. IWGDF guidance on the prevention of foot ulcers in at-risk patients with diabetes. Diabetes Metab Res Rev 2016; 32(Suppl 1):16–24.

42. Myerson M, Papa J, Eaton K, et al. The total-contact cast for management of neuropathic plantar ulceration of the foot. J Bone Joint Surg Am 1992;74(2): 261–9.

43. Armstrong DG, Lavery LA, Kimbriel HR, et al. Activity patterns of patients with diabetic foot ulceration: patients with active ulceration may not adhere to a standard pressure off-loading regimen. Diabetes Care 2003;26(9):2595–7.

44. Addante JB. Metatarsal osteotomy as an office procedure to eradicate intractable plantar keratosis. J Am Podiatry Assoc 1970;60(10):397–9.

45. Helal B. Metatarsal osteotomy for metatarsalgia. J Bone Joint Surg Br 1975;57(2): 187–92.

46. Martin WJ, Weil LS, Smith SD. Surgical management of neurotrophic ulcers in the diabetic foot. J Am Podiatry Assoc 1975;65(4):365–73.

47. Singer A. Surgical treatment of mal perforans. Arch Surg 1976;111(9):964–8.

48. Tamir E, Vigler M, Avisar E, et al. Percutaneous tenotomy for the treatment of diabetic toe ulcers. Foot Ankle Int 2014;35(1):38–43.

49. Cychosz CC, Phisitkul P, Belatti DA, et al. Preventive and therapeutic strategies for diabetic foot ulcers. Foot Ankle Int 2016;37(3):334–43.

50. Haque S, Kakwani R, Chadwick C, et al. Outcome of minimally invasive distal metatarsal metaphyseal osteotomy (DMMO) for lesser toe metatarsalgia. Foot Ankle Int 2016;37(1):58–63.

Minimally Invasive Advances: Lesser Toes Deformities

Guillaume Cordier, MD[a,b,*], Gustavo Araujo Nunes, MD[b,c,1]

KEYWORDS

- Lesser toes deformities • Percutaneous osteotomies • Tenotomy • Forefoot surgery
- Minimally invasive surgery (MIS) • Hammer toe • Claw toe • Toe deformity

KEY POINTS

- Indications are based on clinical examination and analysis of imagery, similar to those for lesser toes minmally invasive surgery.
- As in all percutaneous surgeries, practice requires specific training and respect of learning curve.
- Surgical procedures are adapted to each case, to resulting in à la carte surgery.
- Literature has demonstrated low rates of complications with a minimally invasive surgery (MIS) approach.
- The basic principles of MIS have to be learned and respected to succeed, especially post-operative care with specific bandages for unfixed osteotomies.

INTRODUCTION

Nowadays patients demand fast and painless solutions to treat their pathologies. They also do not accept functional compromise. Despite good published results, open techniques still have improvable functional results.[1,2] To meet the challenge, foot surgeons have had to adapt their procedures. Some have started to practice minimally invasive surgery (MIS) with procedures inspired by podiatric techniques.

Since 2002, the Group of Research and Study in Minimally Invasive Surgery of the Foot (GRECMIP–MIFAS) team has improved and developed procedures to respond these expectations. The goal is triple: to describe anatomic dedicated knowledge for each procedure by anatomic specific research, to improve the understanding of the pathophysiology to clarify indications, and finally to confirm long-term results

Finance: None.

[a] Clinique du Sport Bordeaux-Mérignac, France; [b] GRECMIP-MIFAS (Groupe de Recherche en Chirurgie Mini-Invasive du Pied–Minimally Invasive Foot and Ankle Society), 2 rue Negrevergne, Merignac 33700, France; [c] Hospital Ortopédico, Belo Horizonte, Minas Gerais, Brazil

[1] Present address: Muzambinho street 105/803 - Cruzeiro, Belo Horizonte - Minas Gerais, 30310280 Brazil

* Corresponding author. Clinique du Sport Bordeaux-Mérignac, Chirurgie du Sport - Foot and Ankle, 2 rue negrevergne, Merignac 33700, France.

E-mail address: docteurcordier@yahoo.fr

Foot Ankle Clin N Am 25 (2020) 461–478
https://doi.org/10.1016/j.fcl.2020.05.008
1083-7515/20/
foot.theclinics.com

with patient follow-up and publications. Treatment of lesser toes deformities have evolved during the past decade. The best example is the modification by Piclet-Legré of the team[3] of the flexor tendon tenotomies by a selective tenotomy of the flexor brevis to avoid a floating toe. Currently, MIS procedures to treat lesser toes deformities can be considered a mature technique. Due to their technical versatility and high correction potential, with a low rate of complications, they have become among the main surgeries of percutaneous techniques.[4] Toe deformities are complex clinical entities, resulting from an imbalance between the intrinsic and extrinsic muscles caused by improper shoe wear, trauma, inflammatory arthritis, and neuromuscular, metabolic, and degenerative diseases.[5] These imbalances can lead to a wide variety of deformities, and procedure selection sometimes is difficult. The choice of technique is based on the morphologic and functional criteria assessed by clinical examination.[6,7] The aim is to realign the deformity, preserve or restore the function, and ensure a quicker postoperative recovery. To achieve a good correction of the deformity linked to a good functional result were developed.

Although they seem technically simple procedures, there are important technical details for each of them to obtain a reliable correction and reach success in lesser toes deformity treatment. The philosophy of MIS techniques is to add techniques perioperatively until a perfect reduction of the deformity is reached. Practical training is mandatory before starting the experience; the foot surgeon must learn theoretic and practical aspects to master this à la carte surgery.

GENERALITIES

MIS cannot be performed without training. The goal is to reduce the learning curve and the complications related to the procedure. Principles of percutaneous practice have to be learned, especially about safe anatomic areas for the different procedures. The surgical sequences are identical for all procedures: incisions, creation of the working space, and tenotomies and/or osteotomies. The use of specific devices like percutaneous burrs also requires training in practical courses. MIS practice needs the same preoperative assessment as does open surgery. Percutaneous procedures are like a tool for the foot surgeon. The surgery must be planned, with a clinical examination that details each deformity with localization and type. Even for lesser toes treatment, the gait, posterior muscular chain, and entire foot are observed. The imagery also is analyzed to confirm indications. The authors emphasize that these generalities about MIS are crucial to success.

Positioning

The patient is positioned in a dorsal position with the foot outside the operative table (**Fig. 1**). The position must allow a reliable procedure of the surgeon. The ergonomics to practice is individual and the patient's position can be adapted. The surgical approach can be resulted in medial or lateral to the toes depending on the side of the foot, the dominant hand of the surgeon, and the deformity deviation. Unlike traditional open surgery patient positioning is as important as surgeon positioning to achieve proper ergonomics and correctly perform surgical procedures, including fluoroscopic controls.

Anesthesia

Locoregional anesthesia is the gold standard. There are fewer side effects than with general anesthesia and this type of anesthesia allows better management of early postoperative pain. A purely sensory anesthesia can be used to test per-operatively

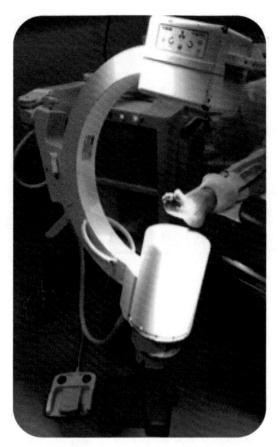

Fig. 1. Positioning.

the result of surgical procedures on the toes deformities, asking the patient to move the toes.

Tourniquet

An ankle tourniquet is not necessary; it could be used if associated procedures require it. The tourniquet presses on the musculature and generates a false modification of the deformities, making it more difficult to evaluate their true passive correction. Furthermore, surgery without tourniquet allows bleeding, which is helpful during the procedure to refresh the burr, reducing burns of bone and soft tissues.

Equipment

Specific equipment is required to practice MIS:

- Beaver blade (**Fig. 2**A): an adapted knife allows resulting in procedures: portals, ligamentous release, arthrotomy, or tenotomies. The smaller size (1 mm) is the gold standard. Some surgeons developed experience with a 3-mm blade.
- Percutaneous instruments
  - Periosteal elevator (**Fig. 2**B): this instrument is necessary to create working space before the use of the burr.

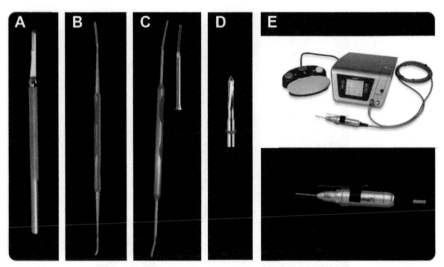

Fig. 2. Specific instruments. (*A*) Beaver blade. (*B*) Periosteal elevator. (*C*) Rasp. (*D*) Shannon burr 8 mm. (*E*) Drill with handpiece.

- o The rasp (**Fig. 2**C) is useful to remove bone paste after bone resection in addition to washing (eg, condylectomy procedure).
- o Percutaneous burr (**Fig. 2**D): to treat lesser toes, the burr's size has to be adapted; the gold standard to perform toe osteotomies is a burr 2-mm × 8-mm (eg, short Shannon, FH ORTHO, Heimsbrunn, France).
- o Drill (**Fig. 2**E): a dedicated low-speed, high-torque drill with a handpiece is required.
- Mini C-arm fluoroscope: this equipment is essential and routinely used to perform percutaneous surgery. Fluoroscopic control has to be performed rigorously with 2 orthogonal incidences. There are concerns about radiation exposure and risks associated with the surgical team. Although it is known that the equivalent annual dose limit for professionally exposed individuals of 20 mSv is unlikely to be achieved by orthopedic surgeons, the use of the mini C-arm instead of the large conventional C-arm is recommended. Some studies have proved that the mini C-arm has been safer and reduces the radiation exposure of the surgeon.[8,9] In addition, the mini C-arm is surgeon operated, has a smaller base area, and is more maneuverable, allowing the required fluoroscopic visualization. Certainly, radiation exposure will have to decrease with time and experience of the surgeon.

Technical note: radiologist education is important to avoid x-ray reports with unadapted comments that may worry the patient (eg, displaced fracture of proximal phalangeal [P1] instead of P1 osteotomy).

- Education of the patient: Due to the absence of pain, immediate post operative full weight bearing combined with the minimal skin incision, some patients tend to neglect basic principles of postoperative care. It is important that surgeons advise patients preoperatively about the importance of postoperative care to obtaining good results. Unrealistic expectations about time to return to activity should be controlled by a preoperative warning. Surgeons should explain that even with MIS with a minimal skin incision and less soft tissue injury, bone and soft tissue procedures take time to heal and demand respect for MIS basic principles in the postoperative period. Also, some steps of postoperative time are specific and can be considered complications by patients if they have not been explained (eg, stains of blood on the dressing).

Classification

To improve surgical planning and scientific reports and to facilitate surgeon communication, lesser toes deformities were standardized with a dedicated international classification proposed by Piclet-Legré[3] that is validated within the French Association of Foot and Ankle surgeons.[10] It is a simple and logical morphologic classification that describes the position of each joint of the toe.

Types of Procedures

Surgical procedures are performed on soft tissue and/or on the bone.

Soft tissue procedures

- Tenotomies: flexors, extensors
- Joint procedure: arthrolysis

Bone procedures

- Extra-articular procedures: phalangeal osteotomies
- Articular procedures: condylectomy and arthroplasty; arthrodesis

Postoperative Care

MIS postoperative care is very peculiar and different compared with open surgery.

Success of percutaneous surgery depends on the postoperative stage, which often is overlooked by some surgeons. This step is considered as a continuation of the surgery. Neglecting the basic rules of MIS, including postoperative care, increases the risk of complications, impairing the final results.

Elevation of the foot and cryotherapy

Edema is part of the postoperative sequence of foot surgery; it may be important in MIS if the osteotomies are unfixed; it is recommended that patients, during the first 7 days after surgery, keep the operated limb elevated between 2 periods of standing. The use of ice, frequently for a short time, also is recommended. The goal is to reduce swelling and therefore pain.

Postoperative footwear and weight bearing

Full weight bearing is allowed in cases of isolated toe treatment, with a postoperative flat shoe for 4 weeks. Of course, according to the associated procedures, this rule can be modified.

Dressings

The dressing is considered one of the most important basic principles of MIS and continuity of surgical treatment, because it is responsible for maintaining the corrections acquired through surgery. Dressing is like an external fixation for unfixed osteotomies. To achieve success in lesser toes percutaneous treatment, it is imperative to follow the principles according to these dressings.

Bandages should be used in the first 4 weeks to 6 weeks, until consolidation of osteotomies and soft tissue healing. After the first bandage in the operative room, it is important to control the correction through a radiographic or fluoroscopic image.

The toes should be immobilized in the opposite position of the initial deformity. According to the most common deformities, usually the metatarsophalangeal joint (MTPJ) is maintained in plantar flexion, proximal interphalangeal joint (PIPJ) and distal interphalangeal joint (DIPJ) in an extension position, and lesser toes in varus toward the hallux (**Figs. 3** A,B and **4**). To avoid maceration, the toes should be separated by a simple gauze. Bandages can never be circular and an excessively over tightening should be avoided to prevent soft tissue damage. Surgeons have to check the distal perfusion, mainly through fingertip coloring. The first dressing could be done with wet woven gauze, strips, and elastic bandage. To avoid bruises, the authors usually do not close the skin, allowing some bleeding in the first postoperative week. Subsequent bandages can be resulted in between 7 days to 15 days. Then, it is possible to use alternative dressings with kinesiology taping, toe splints, or custom-made orthoplastics.

Physiotherapy
Physiotherapy depends on the procedures (especially associated procedures). Patients start physiotherapy at approximately 3 weeks postoperative. Surgeons have to explain instructions and can provide an information sheet on performing maneuvers against scar adhesions, early mobilization, grasping, and physiologic gait. A physiotherapist can be helpful.

Complications
As with any surgical procedure performed to treat lesser toes deformities, some complications are reported: residual misalignment, functional deficit, infection, neurovascular injury, pseudarthrosis, delayed consolidation, and recurrence. These complications rates are very low and the procedure is considered safe. In order to achieve reliability, however, it is essential to respect the basic principles. In cases of noncompliance, specific complications can occur. For example, using the drill at a very high speed, which is not recommended, may lead to thermal bone necrosis and osteotomy healing delay. Lack of irrigation of the skin during osteotomies can cause skin burns and consequent infection. Inadequate control of postoperative bandages can lead to poor finger alignment and surgery failure.

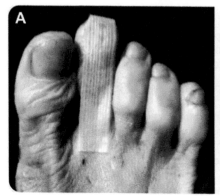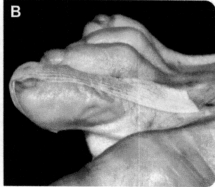

Fig. 3. Bandages to maintain PIPJ extension with adhesive wound closure strips. (*A*) frontal view. (*B*) lateral view.

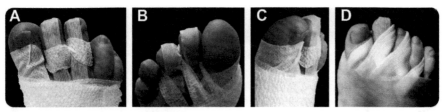

Fig. 4. Bandages to maintain MTPJ flexion. (*A*) Elastic bandage in the frontal view, (*B*) plantar view and (*C*) lateral view. (*D*) Woven gauze.

SOFT TISSUE PROCEDURES
Flexor Digitorum Brevis Tenotomy and Proximal Interphalangeal Joint Arthrolysis

The incision is done on the lateral or medial side of the proximal phalange (P1) (depending on the operated foot and according to the dominant hand of the surgeon), at the level of distal metaphysis (**Fig. 5**). The toe is maintained in plantar flexion during the release to anteriorize and then protect the neurovascular bundle. The beaver blade is introduced directly to the bone and then slipped to the plantar side of P1. The beaver blade progresses distally against the bone condyles and rotates 90° to cut the PIPJ plantar capsule. The next step is to rotate it back and continue the movement distally on the plantar side of the middle phalange (P2), performing the tenotomy of the 2 slips of flexor digitorum brevis (FDB). During this procedure with rotational and axial movement, the beaver blade must keep parallel to the plantar side of P2. A periosteal elevator is introduced to check that a complete section of these slips has been achieved and a PIPJ hyperextension is performed to confirm the adequate release.

Technical note: in cases of rigid deformity of PIPJ, the plantar capsule release achieved by this approach is mandatory to correct rigid deformities presented at this level.

Flexor Digitorum Longus Tenotomy and Distal Interphalangeal Joint Arthrolysis

A longitudinal and plantar incision is performed at the level of DIPJ (**Fig. 6**). The beaver blade is introduced perpendicularly and rotated 90°. With a lateral and/or medial movement, the flexor digitorum longus (FDL) is sectioned. During the release, the toe is simultaneously dorsiflexed, which facilitates the tenotomy and allows the surgeon to feel when it has been completed. Then the beaver blade can be introduced directly to the joint to add a DIPJ arthrolysis.

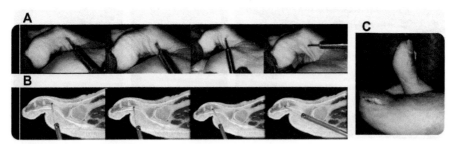

Fig. 5. Tenotomy of flexors brevis. Surgical steps observed in clinical (*A*) and anatomical (*B*) aspects. (*C*) PIPJ hyperextension achieved.

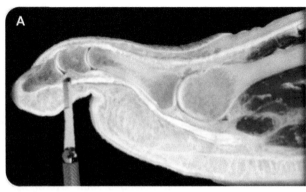
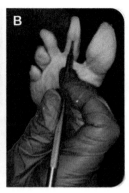

Fig. 6. Flexor longus tenotomy. (*A*) Anatomic view. (*B*) Surgical view.

Flexor Digitorum Brevis and Longus Tenotomies

To achieve both brevis and longus tendon, the incision is performed by a plantar approach of the base of P1 (1 cm distally to MTPJ) (**Fig. 7**). The beaver blade is introduced perpendicularly to the plantar side of P1 and rotates 90°, with a lateral and/or medial movement sectioning both tendons. During the release, the toe should be simultaneously dorsiflexed putting, tension on puting tension on the flexor tendons. A periosteal elevator can be introduced to check that a complete section of these tendons has been achieved. The surgeon can feel the section of the tendons that leads to an increasing of the dorsal flexion of the toe.

Technical note: disadvantages of this technique are obtaining a floating toe and loss of toe grasping movement. The authors advise applying this procedure for rigid deformity of old people with low functional demand.

Extensor Digitorum Tendons Tenotomies and Metatarsophalangeal Arthrolysis

The incision is done at the dorsal side of the MTPJ just above the extensor digitorum longus (EDL), longitudinally and parallel to the tendon to avoid iatrogenic soft tissue damage (nerve and vessels) (**Fig. 8**). At this location, the 2 tendons are close and the extensor digitorum brevis (EDB) runs laterally to the longus. The beaver blade is introduced against the extensor tendon and rotated 90°; a lateral procedure is performed to result in the tenotomy. The surgeon performs a simultaneous plantar flexion of the toe during the beaver blade movement; by the way, at the end of the movement it is possible to feel the full section. Sometimes, the tendon can be seen tensioning by

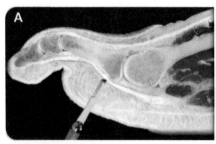
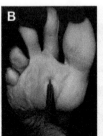
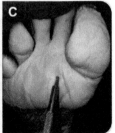

Fig. 7. Flexor longus and brevis tenotomies (*A*) Anatomic view. (*B*) Surgical view: portal. (*C*) Surgical view: cutting both flexor tendons.

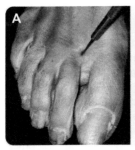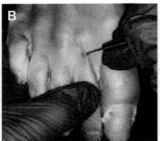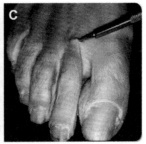

Fig. 8. Extensors tendons tenotomies. (*A*) Approach. (*B*) Rotation of the beaver blade. (*C*) Cutting the tendons.

plantar flexion before the procedure and disappear after the procedure. If MTPJ capsulotomy is indicated, the beaver blade is introduced, deepening inside the joint, and the capsule is sectioned by a mediolateral procedure. Sometimes, due to subluxated MTPJ, it is difficult to access the joint. To facilitate the entry of the Beaver blade inside the joint, a longitudinal traction of the toes can be performed, reducing and opening the joint. Fluoroscopy also can be used to confirm if the beaver blade is in the level of the joint.

Technical notes

- Performing an extensor tenotomy at MTPJ level will maintain the extensor slings connected to the proximal part of the tendon. Due to it, the extensor tendon will not retract proximally and some function will be preserved. (**Fig. 9**).
- The MTPJ arthrolysis generally is required for MP dislocation correction and is the logical deep extension of the extensor tenotomies in cases of extensor tenotomy insufficient to reduce the deformity. Sometimes this dislocation is associated varus or valgus deformity of the toe and in these cases the authors can perform the capsulotomy selectively lateral or medial, according to the deformity. This procedure has the risk of postoperative falling toe due to loss of dorsal stabilizers.

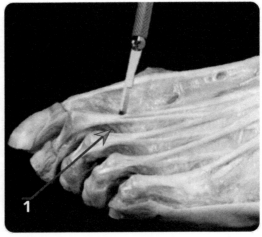

Fig. 9. Red arrow (1) indicating the area of extensor sling, that avoid retraction of the extensor tendons.

BONE PROCEDURES
Proximal Phalangeal Osteotomy

There are some technical variations to result in P1 osteotomy. The portal can be performed through plantar or medial/lateral approach, according to the surgeon preference. The osteotomy can be partial (monocortical) or complete (bicortical), allowing several technical configurations.

Partial osteotomy is more technically demanding than complete osteotomy and preferably is used to correct moderate sagittal deformities and varus or valgus malalignment. Bicortical osteotomy is used to correct other severe and combined deformities, with rotational components, and also to shorten the toe. Bicortical osteotomy also can be done in an oblique direction. This oblique cut can be used to shorten P1, because it is more efficient than a bony removal with a burr.

Technical note: to increase bone resection during complete osteotomy, surgeons have to push the bone against the burr and not the burr against the bone.

Proximal phalangeal osteotomy by plantar approach

The plantar approach is similar to the flexor tenotomy approach, 1 cm distal to the metatarsal head (**Figs. 10**A and **11**). Osteotomy is made at the level of the proximal metaphysis. After the incision, with the nondominant hand, the surgeon holds the toe, maintaining MTPJ in dorsiflexion. The beaver blade is inserted longitudinally, touching the bone; then, a periosteal elevator is introduced around the osteotomy site, creating a working area. Osteotomy is performed with a burr perpendicular to the bone. To result in a bicortical osteotomy, the Shannon burr is inserted through the plantar side of the phalanx, cutting the plantar and dorsal cortex. Using a wrist movement, the burr is rotated in the medial and lateral directions to complete the osteotomy. Another option is to perform the osteotomy from one side to the other side (depending on the foot operated and the dominant hand of the surgeon).

P1 monocortical osteotomy resulted in by a plantar approach usually is used for correct sagittal plane deformity at MTPJ. The goal is to create a dorsal hinge with a plantar closure wedge. The burr is inserted through the middle of the plantar side of the P1. When the burr touches the dorsal cortex, the surgeon must stop and rotate the burr in both medial and lateral directions to complete the osteotomy, always preserving

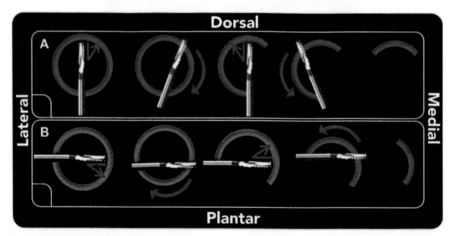

Fig. 10. Monocortical P1 osteotomy steps. (*A*) Creating a plantar closure wedge by a plantar approach. (*B*) Creating a lateral closure wedge by a lateral approach.

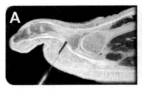
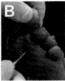
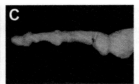

Fig. 11. P1 osteotomy by plantar approach. (*A*) Anatomic view (*B*) Surgical view. (*C*) View of the final aspect on an artificial bone (*D*) Radiographic final aspect.

the dorsal cortex. To facilitate the wedge closure, a dorsolateral and dorsomedial P1 corner also can be carefully and gently cut. To close the wedge, the surgeon performs a smooth reduction maneuver by flexing the distal fragment. If further correction is required, the plantar wedge can be increased, cutting the bottom edge of the bone at the osteotomy level.

Technical note: the osteotomy is done in the proximal metaphysis area of P1 to optimize bone healing and to be as close as possible from the level of deformity. Be careful, the osteotomy should not be made to close to the joint to avoid inadvertent intra-articular fracture. When surgeons introduce the burr, they easily can feel the diaphysis by an anteroposterior movement and find the metaphysis at the inferior part. A fluoroscopic control is advised at the beginning of the practice.

Proximal phalangeal osteotomy by lateral/medial approach

There are 2 options used to perform the lateral approach: midaxial incision and a dorsolateral incision at the proximal metaphyseal level of P1 (or medial/dorsomedial depending on the deformity deviation) (**Fig. 10**B; **Fig. 12**). The beaver blade is inserted longitudinally, touching the bone; then, a periosteal elevator is introduced superiorly and inferiorly, creating a working area in the osteotomy site. With this approach, a monocortical or bicortical osteotomy is performed. Transverse mono-cortical osteotomy used to correct a varus or valgus deformity is approached in the opposite side of the deformity. The access should be done on the contralateral side of the deformity. For example, to correct a medial toe deviation, a lateral closure wedge has to be created, preserving the medial cortex. The burr is introduced into P1 at the proximal metaphysis level preserving the opposite cortex. The subsequent step is result in the osteotomy swepting the burr in dorsal and plantar direction. The contralateral wall is maintained intact and the surgeon can close the osteotomy, making a smooth reduction maneuver. To correct a dorsal toe deviation by a mono-cortical osteotomy, a plantar closure wedge has to be created, preserving the dorsal cortex. According to bicortical osteotomy, the technique is similar to that of a plantar approach.

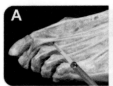
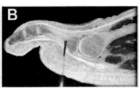
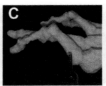
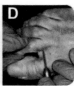

Fig. 12. P1 osteotomy by medial approach. (*A*) Anatomical frontal view. (*B*) Anatomical lateral view. (*C*) View on an artificial bone. (*D*) Surgical view.

Proximal Phalangeal Oblique Osteotomy Technique

The oblique osteotomy is resulted in from distal to proximal. The approach is made distally, by a midaxial lateral incision at the P1 distal metaphyseal-diaphyseal junction.

The burr is introduced perpendicularly at this level and, after touching the bone, the burr is rotated to the required obliquity (generally 45°) in a proximal direction. As described by Redfern and Vernois,[5] the cut is completed in 2 stages. An initial dorsal and plantar sweep of the burr creates the distal half of the osteotomy. The burr then is advanced, and the second part, proximal half of the osteotomy, is completed.

Middle Phalangeal Osteotomy

The approach is performed by a midaxial lateral or medial incision at the diaphyseal level of P2 (metaphysis is too close to the joint) (**Fig. 13**). Like the P1 osteotomies, there are several possibilities, and the osteotomy can be bicortical or monocortical. Monocortical osteotomy allows the correction in the coronal plane by creating a lateral or medial wedge and also in the sagittal plane by a dorsal or plantar wedge. According to the bicortical option, these deformities also can be corrected and the toe shortened. To perform the bicortical osteotomy, the burr is introduced into P2, cutting medial and lateral cortex. Then the burr swept in dorsal and plantar, completing the osteotomy. According to the monocortical option, the P2 dorsiflexion osteotomy commonly is used. By the midaxial incision, the burr is introduced into P2 and swept only to dorsal so that the plantar cortex is maintained and a dorsal wedge is created. The osteotomy is closed by external maneuver.

Condyloplasty and Arthroplasty

The condyloplasty or arthroplasty can be done similarly to the PIPJ and DIPJ (**Fig. 14**). The approach is accomplished through a dorsolateral or dorsomedial incision at the level of the joint. A periosteal elevator is used to create the working space up to the dorsal joint prominences. The Shannon burr is introduced and through a rotational movement against the dorsal part of the bone the prominences are removed. The debris is removed by flushing with saline solution. It is important to highlight that joint washing should be done excessively in order to remove all debris. The bone debris is removed using the specific percutaneous rasps.

If the condyloplasty is not good enough, the surgeon can introduce the burr into the joint and remove the distal part of the head of the proximal phalanx and/or the base of the distal one to result in an arthroplasty.

Arthrodesis

Proximal interphalangeal joint arthrodesis

The surgical approach is done by a midaxial medial or lateral incision at the level of PIPJ. The periosteal elevator is used to create a working space inside the joint. A Shannon burr is inserted into the joint and used to remove the P1 and P2 cartilage

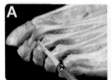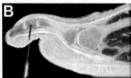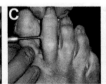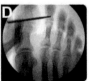

Fig. 13. P2 Osteotomy. (*A*) Anatomic view of the portal. (*B*) Anatomic view of introduction of the burr. (*C*) Surgical view. (*D*) Radiographic view.

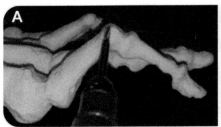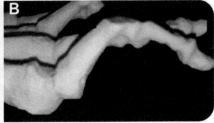

Fig. 14. Condilectomy exemplified in an artificial bone. (*A*) Bone resection using the burr. (*B*) Final result.

to prepare the bone. If more resection is desired, it is possible to apply the respective phalanges against the cutting burr. Through the portal, the debris is removed by flushing with saline solution. The joint can be fixed using 1 intramedullary 1-mm Kirschner (K)-wire (or 2 crossed K-wires).

Distal interphalangeal joint arthrodesis

The surgical approach is done by a midaxial medial or lateral incision at the level of DIPJ. A Shannon burr is inserted into the joint and used to remove the P2 and P3 cartilage to prepare the bone. Fixation also is similar, using 1 intramedullary 1-mm K-wire.

INDICATIONS

Preoperative clinical evaluation is essential to understand each deformity and choose the appropriate surgical technique. The procedures are performed in stages, step by step, according to the correction and reducibility of the deformity evaluated peroperatively. It is important to point out that there are numerous complex deformities and each must be addressed with some specific procedures. The goal is to restore a balance between stabilizers of the toe. The most common indications are discussed.
   The choice of technique is based on morphologic, functional, and etiologic criteria.

- Morphologic criteria: based on each joint sagittal (flexion/extension) and transverse (varus/valgus) plane deformity
- Functional criteria: deformities can be flexible, semirigid, or rigid.
- Etiologic criteria: can guide procedure choice; tenotomies typically are indicated for neurologic cases; P2 isolated osteotomy is performed for clinodactyly; iatrogenic or posttraumatic deformities toes may require phalangeal osteotomies.

Proximal Interphalangeal Joint Flexion Deformity

The PIPJ flexion deformity is the most common deformity of this joint and can be associated with DIPJ and MPJ deformities. This strategy can be applied to correct this deformity.

- FDB tenotomy and PIPJ release are done systematically.
- Plantar flexion P1 osteotomy is added most of the time to complete the reduction. It can correct deformity at the MPJ level and, if extensor tendons are intact and the PIPJ is flexible, then, as the osteotomy is closed, the extensor tendons act on the PIPJ and DIPJ to straighten them.
- P2 osteotomy is performed if there is still a PIPJ flexion deformity after the previous procedures (**Fig. 15**).
- Extensor tenotomy is used when there is a residual MPJ extension deformity.

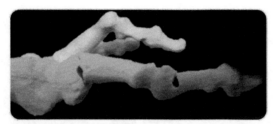

Fig. 15. P1 and P2 partial osteotomies associated with a condylectomy demonstrated in an artificial bone.

Technical notes

- In cases of rigid deformity, some surgeons are more confident using an arthrodesis implant, to avoid a partial result.
- Tenotomies of both flexors are performed only in cases of residual plantar flexion and must be avoided because of poor functional result (floating toe). It could be helpful for older patients with rigid deformities and low functional demand.

Proximal Interphalangeal Joint and Distal Interphalangeal Joint Flexion Deformity

When there is an associated deformity of these the PIPJ and DIPJ, the only difference from treating the isolated PIPJ deformity, described previously, is that instead of performing an FDB tenotomy, FDL tenotomy is performed. The sequence procedures are similar.

- FDL tenotomy is done first.
- P1 osteotomy.
- P2 osteotomy.

Distal Interphalangeal Joint Flexion Deformity

- FDL tenotomy is the first step of the procedure.
- P2 osteotomy is added in cases of residual DIPJ flexion.

Distal Interphalangeal Joint Lateral or Medial Deformity

- P2 osteotomy: especially with a monocortical medial or lateral osteotomy, according to the deviation, is the best option.

Metatarsophalangeal Joint Extension Deformity

- EDL and EDB tenotomy usually are enough for an isolated MPJ extension deformity without PIPJ flexion.
- P1 osteotomy is required if the evaluation of the reduction is imperfect and requires an additional monocortical P1-lowering osteotomy.

Technical note: plantar plate lesion is treated by metatarsal shortening osteotomy. This procedure must be added every time etiology requires it.

Metatarsophalangeal Joint Dorsal Subluxation

- EDL and EDB tenotomy, dorsal MPJ capsule release, and metatarsal osteotomy are indicated to reach the MPJ reduction. Be careful with an MPJ capsule release. This procedure is indicated only in an MPJ subluxation or dislocation; in other situations, it can lead to a partially dislocated and unstable toe if resulted without criteria.

Metatarsophalangeal Joint (Lateral or Medial Subluxation)

- MPJ release and P1 osteotomy can achieve the reduction. This should be considered a palliative procedure and most of the time it is necessary to practice a distal metatarsal osteotomy to shorten the length of the metatarsal and avoid an evolution toward dislocation.

CURRENT BIBLIOGRAPHY

The surgical treatment of lesser toes pathologies has been studied over the years by several investigators.[11–13] Open surgery was considered the gold standard for these deformities, and various procedures, such as tendon transfers, arthroplasty, arthrodesis, and plantar plate repair, have been reported in the literature.[1,12]

Several investigators have published case series of hammer toe treatment by an open approach, with resection arthroplasty of the PIPJ, with intramedullary fixation by a K-wire or other implants and tendon transfers.[11,12,14–16] They had a high satisfaction rates and significant improvement in American Orthopaedic Foot and Ankle Society scores and in good alignment of toes. Nevertheless, they shared some similar complications. Because toe alignment is acquired at the expense of a PIPJ arthrodesis, these patients developed stiffness and functional deficit with loss of toes grasping. Also, soft tissue healing problems and problems with the use of K-wires were observed, including breakage, infection, and pin migration.[11,16–18]

To avoid these complications, percutaneous techniques for the correction of lesser toes began to be developed and studied in Europe. Initially, nonselective percutaneous flexor tendon tenotomies were described for the treatment of finger deformities in patients with diabetic ulcers. Debarge and colleagues[19] described their percutaneous series in 50 patients associating metatarsal osteotomies to FDB and FDL tenotomies to treat claw toe deformity and, despite already enjoying the advantages of the percutaneous pathway, reported 82% satisfaction with minor soft tissue complications. Therefore, the patients in this study still presented, as in the other techniques, functional limitation losing active plantar flexion.[19]

To improve anatomic correction, preserve articular range of motion, and maintain plantar grip of the toes. some technical modifications were developed. One of them, described by a French foot surgeon, Piclet- Legré,[3] includes the selective tenotomy of the flexor tendons. The advantage of this selective tenotomy is to conserve the grasping function of toes, avoiding floating toe. In 2015, Frey and colleagues[1] published their results from a series of 57 feet presenting an isolated second toe PIPJ deformity without metatarsalgia or DIP deformity treated with a selective FDB tenotomy, plantar PIPJ release, and P1 osteotomy. Extensor tenotomy was performed in 42% of cases. Subjective results showed an overall satisfaction rate of 89.5%, 98% for cosmetic results, and 81% for pain relief. Regarding the stiffness, only 12% of the toes were stiff (rigid PIPJ with no passive flexion) and 86% of the toes had preserved active plantar flexion, even though 74% of the toes were preoperatively semirigid or rigid. Only 2 failures (3.5%) were revised with PIPJ fusion.[1]

The literature still has scarce works with higher levels of evidence. The only comparative study between open and percutaneous surgery evaluated hammer toe treatments performed by an open resection arthroplasty of the PIPJ fixed with a K-wire versus a percutaneous approach of proximal phalange osteotomy combined with tendon release of toes wrapped in dressing for 3 weeks. The investigators found equivalent results in terms of correction and patient satisfaction; however, greater

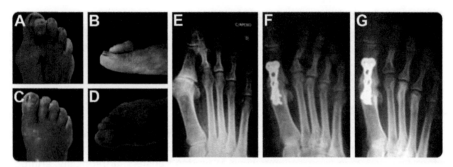

Fig. 16. Clinical case of treatment of second toe deformity associated with hallux rigidus. (*A*) Frontal view and (*B*) lateral view of clinical preoperative aspect. (*C*) Frontal view and (*D*) lateral view of clinical postoperative aspect. (*E*) Radiographic preoperative view. (*F*) Radiographic aspect 3 weeks postoperative and (*G*) 12 weeks postoperative.

infection and recurrence rates were found in the PIPJ arthroplasty resection group. In the other hand the percutaneous group has showed a greater bone consolidation delay, involving approximately 20% of the cases.[20]

Recently, Nieto-García and colleagues,[21] in order to continue improving on studies about functional results after a percutaneous lesser toes deformity correction, published a retrospective study in which they analyzed if the association of tenotomies with incomplete or partial phalanx osteotomies used to treat a reducible deformity of the PIPJ (reducible hammer and claw toe) has a significant impact on the clinical outcomes. They started the correction in 223 patients with an incomplete osteotomy of the P1, always starting from proximal to distal phalanges. After the bone procedure, if the incomplete reducibility of the toe deformity persisted, they added flexor and/or extensor tenotomie. In 129 (57.8%) cases, correction of the deformity by phalangeal incomplete osteotomy without additional tenotomies was performed, and, in 94 (42.2%) cases, it was necessary to combine flexor and/or extensor tenotomies. The investigators concluded that an isolated phalangeal incomplete osteotomy can provide a satisfactory correction of a reducible lesser toes deformity with functional and biomechanical restoration, with a low percentage of complications, and that the addition of flexor/extensor tenotomies enhances the occurrence of adverse events and complications.[21]

CLINICAL CASE

A 69-year-old woman presented with severe crossover second toe, metatarsalgia, and associated hallux rigidus on the right foot. The surgical technique used to treat the lesser toes resulted in the second toe was extensor tenotomy, FDB tenotomy, PIPJ release, and percutaneous transverse P1 osteotomy by a lateral approach. On the third and fourth toes, only the FDB tenotomy was performed. The treatment of the hallux rigidus was resulted by an open fusion of the first MTPJ and the treatment for the metatarsalgia by a distal minimally invasive metatarsal osteotomy of the second, third and fourth metatarsal (**Fig. 16**).

CONFLICT OF INTEREST

The authors declare that they have no conflict of interest.

REFERENCES

1. Frey S, Hélix-Giordanino M, Piclet-Legré B. Percutaneous correction of second toe proximal deformity: proximal interphalangeal release, flexor digitorum brevis tenotomy and proximal phalanx osteotomy. Orthop Traumatol Surg Res 2015; 101(6):753–8.
2. Sergio Fernández C, Wagner E, Ortiz C. Lesser toes proximal interphalangeal joint fusion in rigid claw toes. Foot Ankle Clin 2012;17(3):473–80.
3. Piclet- Legré B. Traitement Chirurgical Percutané Des Déformations Des Orteils Latéraux, Chirurgie mini-invasive Et Percutanée Du Pied. Paris (France): Sauramps médical Ed; 2009. p. 157–67.
4. Shirzad K, Kiesau C, DeOrio J, et al. Lesser toe deformities. J Am Acad Orthop Surg 2011;19(8):505–14.
5. Redfern D, Vernois J. Percutaneous surgery for metatarsalgia and the lesser toes. Foot Ankle Clin 2016;21(3):527–50.
6. Frey-Ollivier S, Catena F, Hélix-Giordanino M, et al. Treatment of flexible lesser toe deformities. Foot Ankle Clin 2018;23(1):69–90.
7. Redfern D, Vernois J, Legré B. Percutaneous surgery of the forefoot. Clin Podiatr Med Surg 2015;32(3):291–332.
8. Gangopadhyay S, Scammell B. Optimising use of the mini C-arm in foot and ankle surgery. Foot Ankle Surg 2009;15(3):139–43.
9. Shoaib A, Rethnam U, Bansal R, et al. A comparison of radiation exposure with the conventional versus mini C arm in orthopedic extremity surgery. Foot Ankle Int 2008;29(1):58–61.
10. Lintz F, Beldame J, Kerhousse G, et al. Intra- and inter-observer reliability of the AFCP classification for sagittal plane deformities of the second toe. Foot Ankle Surg 2019. [Epub ahead of print].
11. Coughlin M, Dorris J, Polk E. Operative repair of the fixed hammertoe deformity. Foot Ankle Int 2000;21(2):94–104.
12. Kramer W, Parman M, Marks R. Hammertoe correction with K-wire fixation. Foot Ankle Int 2015;36(5):494–502.
13. Nery C, Coughlin M, Baumfeld D, et al. Lesser metatarsophalangeal joint instability: prospective evaluation and repair of plantar plate and capsular insufficiency. Foot Ankle Int 2012;33(4):301–11.
14. Basile A, Albo F, Via A. Intramedullary fixation system for the treatment of hammertoe deformity. J Foot Ankle Surg 2015;54(5):910–6.
15. Coillard J, Petri G, van Damme G, et al. Stabilization of proximal interphalangeal joint in lesser toe deformities with an angulated intramedullary implant. Foot Ankle Int 2014;35(4):401–7.
16. O'Kane C, Kilmartin T. Review of proximal interphalangeal joint excisional arthroplasty for the correction of second hammer toe deformity in 100 cases. Foot Ankle Int 2005;26(4):320–5.
17. Lehman D, Smith R. Treatment of symptomatic hammertoe with a proximal interphalangeal joint arthrodesis. Foot Ankle Int 1995;16(9):535–41.
18. Errichiello C, Marcarelli M, Pisani P, et al. Treatment of dynamic claw toe deformity flexor digitorum brevis tendon transfer to interosseous and lumbrical muscles: a literature survey. Foot Ankle Surg 2012;18(4):229–32.
19. Debarge R, Philippot R, Viola J, et al. Clinical outcome after percutaneous flexor tenotomy in forefoot surgery. Int Orthop 2009;33(5):1279–82.

20. Yassin M, Garti A, Heller E, et al. Hammertoe correction with K-wire fixation compared with percutaneous correction. Foot Ankle Spec 2016; 10(5):421–7.
21. Nieto-García E, Ferrer-Torregrosa J, Ramírez-Andrés L, et al. The impact of associated tenotomies on the outcome of incomplete phalangeal osteotomies for lesser toe deformities. J Orthop Surg Res 2019;14(1):308.

Role of Minimally Invasive Surgery in Adult Flatfoot Deformity

Alessio Bernasconi, MD, PhD, FEBOT[a,b],
Robbie Ray, MB ChB, ChM(T&O), FRCSed(T&O), FEBOT[c,*]

KEYWORDS

- Flatfoot • Adult • Tibialis posterior • Minimally invasive • MIS

KEY POINTS

- There are still unanswered questions with regards to the best management of early stages of adult acquired flatfoot deformity (AAFD).
- Minimally invasive surgical techniques can be used in the treatment of flexible AAFD, including tibialis posterior tendoscopy, subtalar arthroereisis, minimally invasive calcaneal osteotomy, and medial proximal gastrocnemius recession.
- Although generally leading to a satisfactory outcome, robust evidence comparing minimally invasive surgery and traditional approaches is still lacking.

INTRODUCTION

Adult acquired flatfoot deformity (AAFD) as a consequence of posterior tibial tendon dysfunction (PTTD) was first classified in 1989 by Johnson and Strom[1] into 3 distinct stages. The first stage was described as inflammation of the posterior tibial tendon. In the second stage, this was accompanied by a flexible flatfoot deformity, and in the third stage, the flatfoot deformity was fixed with hindfoot arthritis. A fourth stage is commonly attributed to Myerson[2] and is described as subsequent valgus ankle osteoarthritis. The treatment of fixed deformities is relatively straightforward with options limited to double or triple hindfoot arthrodesis for stage III disease with the addition of an ankle fusion or ankle replacement for stage IV disease. In earlier stages, however, with a flexible flatfoot, as the understanding of the complex nature of the deformities present in AAFD has increased, so has the push to develop modern

Funded by: CRUI2020.
[a] Department of Public Health, Trauma and Orthopaedics, University of Naples Federico II, Via Pansini 5, Naples 80131, Italy; [b] Foot and Ankle Unit, Royal National Orthopaedic Hospital, Brockley Hill, Stanmore HA7 4LP, UK; [c] Princess Royal University Hospital, King's College Hospital NHS Foundation Trust, Orpington, London BR68ND, UK
* Corresponding author.
E-mail address: robbie1ray1@gmail.com

Foot Ankle Clin N Am 25 (2020) 479–491
https://doi.org/10.1016/j.fcl.2020.05.007
1083-7515/20/© 2020 Elsevier Inc. All rights reserved.

foot.theclinics.com

treatment strategies to address these pathologic conditions.[3] In 2007, Bluman and colleagues[4] published a more detailed classification of PTTD considering the myriad of deformities that contribute toward AAFD (**Table 1**). In their article, they mention that there is a range of surgical alternatives based on the different subcategories, but that many of these were new and they were therefore unfamiliar with all the available techniques and uncertain of the best alternative. The aim of this article is to describe and review the evidence available for minimally invasive surgical techniques that can be used in the treatment of flexible AAFD, including tibialis posterior tendoscopy, subtalar arthroereisis (STA), minimally invasive calcaneal osteotomy, and medial proximal gastrocnemius recession (MPGR).

TIBIALIS POSTERIOR TENDOSCOPY
Background

In Johnson and Strom's original classification, the management of recalcitrant posterior tibial (PT) tendon dysfunction (PTTD stage I) was open synovectomy followed by a period of immobilization.[1] However, in 1995 Wertheimer and colleagues[5] documented a case of a patient affected by posterior tibial tenosynovitis resistant to conservative treatment that was treated through a tendoscopic approach with complete relief of symptoms thereafter. Subsequently, the tendoscopic technique described by van Dijk and Kort[6] has been used as the basis of modern tendoscopic surgery. Upon review of the current literature, the main indication for PT tendoscopy is in the treatment of stage I and stage II PTTD resistant to nonsurgical treatment.[7–12] Through this approach, investigators have been able to assess the status of the tendon and of the near spring ligament and to perform simultaneously tendon synovectomy, vincula resection, debridement of scar, adhesiolysis, and longitudinal tendon tear sutures.[6–11,13]

General Points on Technique

Two small portals placed along the PT tendon 2 cm distally and 2 cm proximally to the malleolar tip, respectively, are sufficient to perform a tendoscopy (**Fig. 1**). A 2.7-mm 30° arthroscope introduced into the tendon sheath enables evaluation of the tendon (**Fig. 2**), and a 4-mm or 2.7-mm arthroscopic synovial resector may be used to debride what is needed (see **Fig. 2**). A classification of spring ligament lesions through this approach has been recently reported,[11] but so far no study has documented its validity in the clinical scenario. A repair of the ligament has also been documented, although this is technically demanding.[14] Postoperatively, no immobilization is required with investigators documenting recovery of full weight-bearing from 2 days to 3 weeks.[6–9,11] Only a few complications have been reported so far, such as inadvertent introduction into the flexor digitorum longus (FDL) tendon sheath[6] and skin discomfort,[9] with no consequences. When patients are counseled, they should be made aware of the risk of failure to relieve their symptoms and the necessity to perform further traditional surgery.[11,12]

SUBTALAR ARTHROEREISIS
Background

Although there is a paucity of good evidence in the English orthopedic literature, STA is a commonly used procedure for AAFD in podiatric circles and in Europe.[15,16] The term *arthroereisis* originates from Greek roots arthro- (joint) and -ereisis (to sustain or support) and describes a procedure finalized to restore the longitudinal medial arch of the foot acting as a support under the subtalar joint, but without fusing

Table 1
Bluman classification of first 2 stages adult acquired flatfoot deformity and relative treatment adopting minimally invasive surgery techniques

Stage	Substage	Main Clinical Findings	Main Radiographic Findings	Suggested Surgical Options After Failure of Conservative Treatment
I	Ia	Tenderness along PTT (underlying systemic inflammatory disease)	Normal	STA + PT tendoscopic synovectomy
	Ib	Tenderness along PTT	Normal	STA + PT tendoscopic synovectomy ± mini-open repair of tendon tear
	Ic	Tenderness along PTT Supple hindfoot valgus (<5°)	Slight hindfoot valgus	MIS calcaneal osteotomy + STA + PT tendoscopic synovectomy ± mini-open repair of tendon tear
II	IIa	Supple hindfoot valgus, forefoot varus	Hindfoot valgus Meary line disrupted Reduced calcaneal pitch	MIS calcaneal osteotomy + STA + PT tendoscopic synovectomy ± FDL transfer and SL augmentation ± Cotton osteotomy
	IIb	Supple hindfoot valgus, forefoot abduction	Hindfoot valgus Talonavicular uncovering Forefoot abduction	MIS calcaneal osteotomy + STA + PT tendoscopic synovectomy ± FDL transfer and SL augmentation
	IIc	Supple hindfoot valgus, fixed forefoot varus, medial column instability	Hindfoot valgus First TMTJ plantar gapping	MIS calcaneal osteotomy + STA + PT tendoscopic synovectomy ± FDL transfer and SL augmentation + MIS Lapidus fusion

Procedures have been listed in the order they are generally performed.
Abbreviations: MIS, minimally invasive surgery; PT, posterior tibial; PTT, posterior tibial tendon; SL, spring ligament; TMTJ, tarsometatarsal joint.

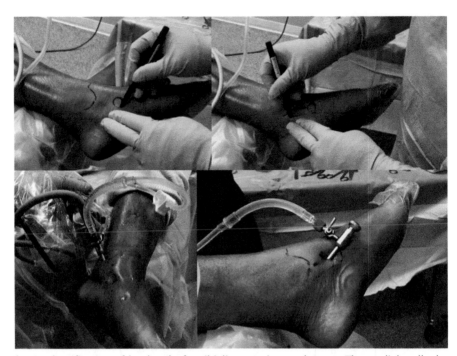

Fig. 1. Identification of landmarks for tibialis posterior tendoscopy. The medial malleolus, the medial tuberosity of navicular (*left upper image*), and the projection of the tibialis posterior tendon (*right upper image*) are defined. After placing the 2 portals (see the text), the access to the tendon can be performed from proximal (*left lower image*) or from distal (*right lower image*). (François Lintz, MD MSc FEBOT, Saint-Jean, France.)

it.[16,17] As per Vogler's classification,[18] 3 types of implants have been described so far: axis-altering, impact-blocking (ie, calcaneo-stop), and self-locking devices (ie, conical or cylindrical implants introduced through the sinus into the canalis tarsi). Although the use of STA was originally introduced for the treatment of pediatric flatfoot, various investigators have reported satisfactory results in the adult population. In particular, STA has been advocated for the treatment of AAFD from stage I to IIc, both as a standalone and as an adjunctive procedure.[9,17,19–21] In a recent article, Walley and colleagues[19] compared 30 feet treated with medializing calcaneal osteotomy, FDL transfer, spring ligament repair, and Achilles tendon lengthening for AAFD against 15 feet that had the same procedure but with additional STA. The investigators found good clinical outcomes in both groups, but STA enabled the achievement of better radiographic correction.[19]

General Points on Technique

The senior author (R.R.) prefers to use a self-locking conical STA implant (ProStop Arthroereisis Subtalar Implant, Arthrex, Naples, FL, USA). The patient is positioned in the floppy lateral position allowing ease of surgery and easy conversion to a supine position for radiographs and subsequent tendoscopy.[22] A 2.5-cm incision is made directly over the sinus tarsi, and sharp dissection is used to visualize the lateral process of the talus. This step is crucial to avoid compressing the fatty contents of the sinus tarsi leading to impingement pain. Progressive trials are inserted until the

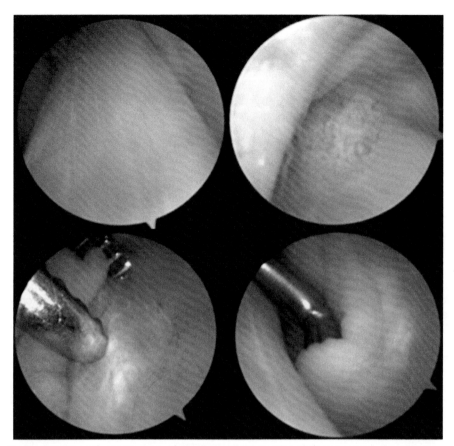

Fig. 2. Examples of visualization of tibialis posterior tendon (*left upper image*) with a synovial loose fragment (*right upper image*) during tendoscopy. The procedure allows the removal of inflamed tissue (*left lower image*) and tests the integrity of spring ligament (*right lower image*). (François Lintz, MD MSc FEBOT, Saint-Jean, France.)

hindfoot is corrected to neutral alignment. In order to avoid overcorrection, a lateral fluoroscopic view of the hindfoot may be taken that will reveal excessive opening of the subtalar joint, suggesting an oversized implant. The STA is then inserted under an image intensifier until the lateral border of the implant is slightly medial to the lateral edge of the talar neck (**Fig. 3**).[16,17] Radiographically, this will correct the talar declination and abduction. The wound is closed with absorbable sutures.

MINIMALLY INVASIVE CALCANEAL OSTEOTOMY
Background

Johnson and Strom's original classification[1] was strongly biased toward disease in the posterior tibial tendon, and for stage II disease, they suggested an FDL transfer. Myerson and colleagues[23] noted that stage II disease was commonly associated with a flexible valgus heel, and when the FDL transfer was performed in isolation, there was frequently residual symptoms and progression of disease. To counteract this, they started to perform a medial slide calcaneal osteotomy. The investigators subsequently published results showing better outcomes with the addition of the osteotomy

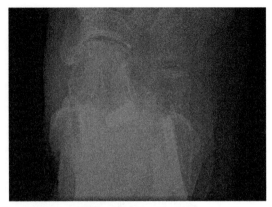

Fig. 3. Postoperative radiograph (dorsoplantar view) showing the positioning of a self-locking implant. Ideally, the proximal extremity should be just medial to the lateral border the talar neck and its tip approximately at the midline of the bone.

in patients with a flexible valgus heel.[23,24] As the understanding of the underlying deformities has improved, it is better understood that a medial slide calcaneal osteotomy is an integral part of correcting frontal plane hindfoot deformity with heel valgus.[25] Open medial slide calcaneal osteotomy is routinely performed through a direct lateral open approach but is associated with a non-negligible rate of wound complication and sural nerve injury. Furthermore, achieving an adequate translation might be technically difficult due to the tension on the soft tissues, which requires generous soft tissue stripping.[26,27] Over the last few years, evidence has emerged showing that a minimally invasive medial slide calcaneal osteotomy is equally effective but with lower complication rates.[28,29] As well as retrospective clinical evidence, cadaveric studies have shown that, when performed correctly, the risk to neurovascular structures is low.[30,31]

General Points on Technique

The patient is positioned in the floppy lateral position.[22] This position allows for the Strayer procedure, calcaneal osteotomy, fixation, and subsequent STA implant all to be performed in the lateral position, which is technically easier, and for the leg to be positioned supine for medial procedures. The foot is positioned so that a true lateral of the calcaneus is seen on imaging. A large guide wire, usually ones used for the screws for fixation will suffice, is used to mark the plane of the osteotomy, which is centered over the calcaneal tuberosity. The wire is also used to mark the mid axial plane of the calcaneus. The crossing of these 2 lines is the ideal starting point for the osteotomy and is where a 5-mm skin incision is made. The wire is then inserted subcutaneously in line with the vertical mark and is used as a cutting block and to ensure there is no risk of straying toward the sural nerve and subtalar joint. A periosteal elevator is used to adequately reflect soft tissues from the lateral surface of the calcaneus. A 3/20-mm irrigated, motorized burr is then inserted through the incision over an open mosquito forceps (to protect the sural nerve). The burr is pushed deep through both cortices and can be felt by the nonoperating hand on the medial side of the calcaneus. The burr is then drawn back because the first stage of the osteotomy is to cut the dorsal and lateral walls leaving the medial wall intact. As the wrist is supinated and the hand is rotated in a plantar direction, the burr cuts through the dorsomedial corner and can again be felt with the nonoperating hand. A check radiograph can be useful to ensure that the plane of the osteotomy is matching the subcutaneous guidewire. The burr is rotated back to the incision site ensuring that the dorsal and lateral walls are fully released. The same technique is used again for the plantar wall and plantar lateral wall. At this point, a check radiograph should reveal an oblique line in the plane of the osteotomy; nevertheless, the bony fragments will be immobile because the medial wall is still intact. The burr is now positioned at the dorsomedial corner, and the osteotomy is used as a cutting block to complete the osteotomy through the medial wall using the nonoperating hand to ensure that the burr does not stray deep and put the medial structures at risk. When the osteotomy is completed, the calcaneus is mobile, and the osteotomy line disappears on radiographs as the calcaneus naturally shortens into the gap. If there is still some small connection of bone and the osteotomy will not easily mobilize, a small laminar spreader can used through the incision to crack these final bridges, which are most commonly on the near, lateral wall because this region is the most difficult to cut. Two guide wires are then inserted into the tuberosity above and below and parallel to the horizontal mark. The surgeon then reduces the osteotomy into neutral with finger pressure, and the assistant drives the wires across the osteotomy. An axial view of the calcaneus can confirm correction. If suitable correction is not achieved, there are 2 ways to improve it. First, a periosteal elevator can be used to forcibly move the calcaneus further; however, the senior author prefers to draw the reduction wires back and reinsert them with a varus tilt, thereby causing a translational and angular correction. Two large compression screws (**Fig. 4**) are then inserted across the osteotomy, and the wound is closed with absorbable sutures.

MEDIAL PROXIMAL GASTROCNEMIUS RELEASE
Background

There is a reasonably convincing scientific basis that a relationship between gastrocnemius-soleus tightness and AAFD exists.[32–34] It is clinically evident that patients who present with symptomatic AAFD frequently have a degree of equinus

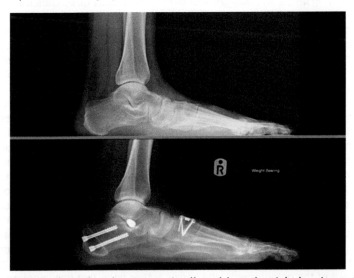

Fig. 4. Preoperative (*upper*) and postoperative (*lower*) lateral weight-bearing radiographs showing minimally invasive surgery flatfoot correction. No proximal displacement of the calcaneal posterior tuberosity is observed, and the metalwork (calcaneal screws, arthroereisis implant, and dorsal cuneiform plate) appear properly positioned.

contracture, and this affects not only dorsiflexion of the ankle but also version and rotation of the subtalar joint, thereby contributing to the deformity.[32,34] Management of equinus contracture can be via Achilles tendon lengthening or gastrocnemius recession. Although these procedures are commonly performed, they require a lengthy period of rehabilitation and can significantly weaken the action of the superficial posterior compartment.

An MPGR is a procedure popularized by Louis Samuel Barouk,[35] who switched from performing a release of both the lateral and the medial gastrocnemius fascia to releasing only the medial fascia in 2005. He found that the overall clinical results were similar with a reduction to almost no complications. In 2012, Abbassian and colleagues[36] reported a series of patients who had an MPGR for recalcitrant plantar fasciitis. In patients who had at least 12 months of symptomatic plantar fasciitis and a positive Silfverskiold test, an isolated MPGR was performed under local anesthetic. In patients with a positive Silfverskiold test, the senior author routinely performs an MPGR when performing an STA or PT tendoscopy.

General Points on Technique

The patient is under general anesthesia and positioned in the recovery position.[37] This position gives excellent access to the area, avoiding the risks of a full prone position. No tourniquet is used because bleeding is minimal, and it is best to cauterize any small bleeders before closing. The medial dimple of the popliteal fossa is marked, and simple square draping is performed. The incision site is marked 1 cm lateral and distal to the crease (**Fig. 5**). The reason for this is to avoid branches of the saphenous vein, which can bleed profusely in the postoperative period and lead to significant hematoma. A horizontal skin incision is used because this heals well in line with the skin crease. Finger dissection is used to deepen the incision to the superficial fascia, and this is incised longitudinally to avoid branches of vessels and nerves. A curved forceps is then used to deliver the medial head of gastrocnemius into the wound, and only the overlying fascia is released under direct vision (see **Fig. 5**). Care must be taken not to damage the hamstring tendons, which can be inadvertently delivered into the wound. Only the skin is closed with absorbable sutures, and a small waterproof dressing is applied. If further surgery is required, the patient is repositioned. If the theater staff is experienced, they can do this while the operating team remains scrubbed.

AUTHORS' ALGORITHM AND TIPS

When using Bluman's more in-depth classification,[4] the senior author uses tendoscopic debridement for stage Ia and Ib in addition to a STA implant with the aim to reduce long-term tendon overloading.[9] Furthermore, in stage Ib, where the tendon inflammation is associated with a split tear, this can be either debrided tendoscopically or repaired through an additional 2-cm incision if more than 50% of the tendon is torn.[9] In stage Ic and IIa, which are accompanied by slight or supple hindfoot valgus, the procedures are accompanied by a minimally invasive medial slide calcaneal osteotomy (**Table 2**). In the authors' experience, a dorsal proximal to plantar distal oblique osteotomy is more technically straightforward than a chevron osteotomy and avoids any risk to the neurovascular structures. Although some may argue that a chevron osteotomy[38] would reduce the risk of a "Mitchell effect" (with proximal displacement of the osteotomy[39]), the senior author finds that this is not an issue as long as a lengthening procedure of the posterior compartment is performed before osteotomy. In order to avoid issues with positioning related to MPGR procedure (patient needs to be placed three-quarters prone for an MPGR and then turned lateral or

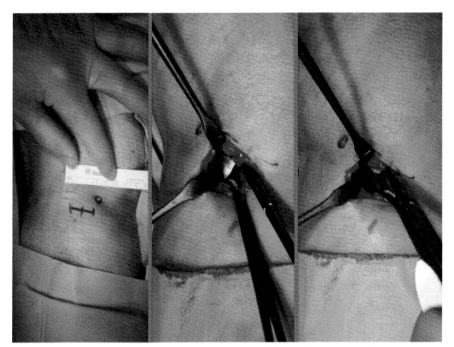

Fig. 5. Some steps of posteromedial gastrocnemius release. Skin marking (*left*), exposition of the medial head of gastrocnemius fascia (*middle*), and splitting of fascia with stretching of the muscle can be stretched (*right*).

floppy lateral for a calcaneal osteotomy), the senior author performs a Strayer procedure from a posterolateral approach before performing the calcaneal osteotomy. The patient is appropriately positioned for this procedure, and because the sural nerve can be seen in the incision and protected, a full release can be easily performed. Of note, in cases whereby PT tendoscopy reveals a severely degenerated tendon, investigators recommend a traditional FDL transfer with spring ligament repair and augmentation with Internal Brace (Arthrex). To the best of the authors' knowledge, it is still unclear at exactly which stage in the disease process medial reconstructive procedures are required compared with when tendon debridement and biomechanical correction of position will suffice. Also, in Bluman stage IIb disease, frequently a medial column procedure is required to plantarflex the first ray. If there is concomitant hallux valgus deformity, the senior author uses a minimally invasive Lapidus procedure and corrects the supination through this. If not, his preference is a dorsal open wedge plantarflexion osteotomy of the medial cuneiform (Cotton) because this is stable and allows weight-bearing at 4 weeks, whereas a minimally invasive plantar closing wedge osteotomy would be unstable on weight-bearing and would necessitate a longer period of non-weight-bearing. In this scenario, the only indication the senior author has for isolated STA is a patient who has been successfully managed with conservative measures but who has pain when not wearing corrective insoles and is unable to maintain a good quality of life and repertoire of shoe wear.

Postoperatively, after STA, the patient is allowed to mobilize fully weight-bearing as tolerated in a boot. When MPGR is performed in isolation or with STA and PT tendoscopy, immediate full weight-bearing mobilization is possible in a boot for 2 weeks followed by physiotherapy and orthotics. When a calcaneal osteotomy is performed (with

Table 2 Technical tips	
Procedure	**Authors' Suggestions**
Tibialis posterior tendoscopy	1. Mark distal portal on awake patient as easier to palpate when muscle contracted 2. Make 0.5-cm mini-open incision through skin and fascia to ease scope entry 3. Use least aggressive, low radius shaver possible as small working space. The senior author prefers a 4-mm Arthrex Torpedo shaver 4. Make proximal portal using light from scope. Usual extent is at posterior medial malleolus 5. If needed, use 2-cm incision for mini-open repair
Subtalar arthroereisis	1. Make 2.5-cm incision over sinus tarsi and make incision through sinus tarsi fat down to bone. This stops soft tissue being forced into the tract 2. Push entry wire anterolateral to posteromedial, should find an easy passage through sinus tarsi 3. Pop through medial skin. This keeps the wire in place during obturator trials 4. Trial 7, 8, and 9 size in order to create working space. Correct size corrects hindfoot and feels solid on insertion. Allow some residual eversion to avoid overcorrection 5. Use dorsoplantar foot medial oblique to assess adequate insertion. Should be 50% under talus with lateral edge of implant medial to the lateral edge of talus. With mini-open approach described, this can be assessed visually also
Minimally invasive calcaneal osteotomy	1. Ensure fluoroscopic true lateral view of calcaneus. This may be better appreciated in the lateral position with the heel further elevated on a dish as compared with the forefoot 2. Mark osteotomy line and mid axial line as described and use a 2-mm wire anteriorly to protect subtalar joint 3. If correction is inadequate, use a small laminar spreader through incision to release soft tissues and a periosteal elevator 4. Insert wires posteriorly in tuberosity fragment without crossing the osteotomy line, then perform correction and ask assistant to advance wires into calcaneal body while maintaining correction
Medial proximal gastrocnemius recession	1. Mark patient while awake because it is much easier to palpate medial popliteal dimple 2. Use a horizontal skin crease incision along Langer lines but a vertical fascial incision 3. Intraoperative coagulation greatly reduces postoperative hematoma, therefore no need of tourniquet

or without Strayer procedure), the patient is immobilized non-weight-bearing in a cast for 4 weeks followed by boot mobilization and physiotherapy.

The aforementioned protocol has been adopted by the senior author since 2018. Out of 5 patients followed at more than 12 months of follow-up, of which 3 had a simple synovectomy and debridement and 2 had a mini-open tendon repair, all patients have been satisfied with the procedure, and no reintervention has been required so far.

SUMMARY

There are still unanswered questions with regards to the best management of early stages of AAFD. Multiple bony and soft tissue procedures have been described so far, and some of them may be performed either through traditional open approach or in a minimally invasive fashion. However, to the best of the authors' knowledge, clear evidence about the superiority of open versus minimally invasive surgical techniques is missing. As described in this article, there is emerging evidence for focusing on lateral correction and medial tendoscopic debridement; nevertheless, further work is required to clarify when formal medial procedures, such as tendon transfers and spring ligament reconstructions, are required. Currently, the senior author uses these procedures if there is MRI evidence of significant tendon disease or a spring ligament tear.

DISCLOSURE

The authors have nothing to disclose.

REFERENCES

1. Johnson KA, Strom DE. Tibialis posterior tendon dysfunction. Clin Orthop Relat Res 1989;239:196–206. Available at: http://www.ncbi.nlm.nih.gov/pubmed/2912622.
2. Myerson MS. Adult acquired flatfoot deformity: treatment of dysfunction of the posterior tibial tendon. J Bone Joint Surg 1996;78A:780–92.
3. Abousayed MM, Tartaglione JP, Rosenbaum AJ, et al. Classifications in brief: Johnson and Strom classification of adult-acquired flatfoot deformity. Clin Orthop Relat Res 2016;474(2):588–93.
4. Bluman EM, Title CI, Myerson MS. Posterior tibial tendon rupture: a refined classification system. Foot Ankle Clin 2007;12(2):233–49, v.
5. Wertheimer SJ, Weber CA, Loder BG, et al. The role of endoscopy in treatment of stenosing posterior tibial tenosynovitis. J Foot Ankle Surg 1995;34(1):15–22.
6. van Dijk CN, Kort NSP. Tendoscopy of the posterior tibial tendon. Arthroscopy 1997;13(6):692–8. Available at: https://www.ncbi.nlm.nih.gov/pubmed/9442321.
7. Chow HT, Chan KB, Lui TH. Tendoscopic debridement for stage I posterior tibial tendon dysfunction. Knee Surg Sports Traumatol Arthrosc 2005;13(8):695–8.
8. Bulstra GH, Olsthoorn PGM, Niek van Dijk C. Tendoscopy of the posterior tibial tendon. Foot Ankle Clin 2006;11(2):421–7, viii.
9. Khazen G, Khazen C. Tendoscopy in stage I posterior tibial tendon dysfunction. Foot Ankle Clin 2012;17(3):399–406.
10. Hua Y, Chen S, Li Y, et al. Arthroscopic treatment for posterior tibial tendon lesions with a posterior approach. Knee Surg Sports Traumatol Arthrosc 2015; 23(3):879–83.
11. Bernasconi A, Sadile F, Welck M, et al. Role of tendoscopy in treating stage II posterior tibial tendon dysfunction. Foot Ankle Int 2018;39(4):433–42.
12. Bernasconi A, Sadile F, Smeraglia F, et al. Tendoscopy of Achilles, peroneal and tibialis posterior tendons: an evidence-based update. Foot Ankle Surg 2018; 24(5):374–82.

13. Gianakos AL, Ross KA, Hannon CP, et al. Functional outcomes of tibialis posterior tendoscopy with comparison to magnetic resonance imaging. Foot Ankle Int 2015;36(7):812–9.

14. Lui TH. Endoscopic repair of the superficial deltoid ligament and spring ligament. Arthrosc Tech 2016;5(3):e621–5.

15. Metcalfe SA, Bowling FL, Reeves ND. Subtalar joint arthroereisis in the management of pediatric flexible flatfoot: a critical review of the literature. Foot Ankle Int 2011;32(12):1127–39.

16. Bernasconi A, Lintz F, Sadile F. The role of arthroereisis of the subtalar joint for flatfoot in children and adults. EFORT Open Rev 2017;2(11):438–46.

17. Schon LC. Subtalar arthroereisis: a new exploration of an old concept. Foot Ankle Clin 2007;12(2):329–39.

18. Vogler HM. Subtalar joint blocking operations for pathological pronation syndromes. In: McGlamry ED, editor. Comprehensive textbook of foot surgery. Baltimore: Williams & Wilkins; 1987. p. 447–65.

19. Walley KC, Greene G, Hallam J, et al. Short- to mid-term outcomes following the use of an arthroereisis implant as an adjunct for correction of flexible, acquired flatfoot deformity in adults. Foot Ankle Spec 2019;12(2):122–30.

20. Yasui Y, Tonogai I, Rosenbaum AJ, et al. Use of the arthroereisis screw with tendoscopic delivered platelet-rich plasma for early stage adult acquired flatfoot deformity. Int Orthop 2017;41(2):315–21.

21. Zhu Y, Xu X. Treatment of stage II adult acquired flatfoot deformity with subtalar arthroereises. Foot Ankle Spec 2015;8(3):194–202.

22. Lees D, Rankin KS, Marriott A, et al. Floppy lateral position: technique tip. Foot Ankle Int 2013;34(10):1460–3.

23. Myerson MS, Corrigan J, Thompson F, et al. Tendon transfer combined with calcaneal osteotomy for treatment of posterior tibial tendon insufficiency: a radiological investigation. Foot Ankle Int 1995;16(11):712–8.

24. Myerson MS, Corrigan J. Treatment of posterior tibial tendon dysfunction with flexor digitorum longus tendon transfer and calcaneal osteotomy. Orthopedics 1996;19(5):383–8. Available at: http://www.ncbi.nlm.nih.gov/pubmed/8727331. Accessed September 20, 2019.

25. Guha AR, Perera AM. Calcaneal osteotomy in the treatment of adult acquired flatfoot deformity. Foot Ankle Clin 2012;17(2):247–58.

26. Complications of calcaneal osteotomy Ray R., Jameson S., and Kumar S. Orthopaedic Proceedings 2010 92-B:SUPP_IV, 590-590.

27. Tennant JN, Carmont M, Phisitkul P. Calcaneus osteotomy. Curr Rev Musculoskelet Med 2014;7(4):271–6.

28. Kendal AR, Khalid A, Ball T, et al. Complications of minimally invasive calcaneal osteotomy versus open osteotomy. Foot Ankle Int 2015;36(6):685–90.

29. Kheir E, Borse V, Sharpe J, et al. Medial displacement calcaneal osteotomy using minimally invasive technique. Foot Ankle Int 2015;36(3):248–52.

30. Durston A, Bahoo R, Kadambande S, et al. Minimally invasive calcaneal osteotomy: does the Shannon burr endanger the neurovascular structures? A cadaveric study. J Foot Ankle Surg 2015;54(6):1062–6.

31. Jowett CRJ, Rodda D, Amin A, et al. Minimally invasive calcaneal osteotomy: a cadaveric and clinical evaluation. Foot Ankle Surg 2016;22(4):244–7.

32. Meszaros A, Caudell G. The surgical management of equinus in the adult acquired flatfoot. Clin Podiatr Med Surg 2007;24(4):667–85, viii.

33. Arangio GA, Wasser T, Rogman A. The use of standing lateral tibial-calcaneal angle as a quantitative measurement of Achilles tendon contracture in adult acquired flatfoot. Foot Ankle Int 2006;27(9):685–8.
34. DiGiovanni CW, Langer P. The role of isolated gastrocnemius and combined Achilles contractures in the flatfoot. Foot Ankle Clin 2007;12(2):363–79, viii.
35. Barouk P. Technique, indications, and results of proximal medial gastrocnemius lengthening. Foot Ankle Clin 2014;19(4):795–806.
36. Abbassian A, Kohls-Gatzoulis J, Solan MC. Proximal medial gastrocnemius release in the treatment of recalcitrant plantar fasciitis. Foot Ankle Int 2012; 33(1):14–9.
37. Gougoulias N, Dawe EJC, Sakellariou A. The recovery position for posterior surgery of the ankle and hindfoot. Bone Joint J 2013;95-B(10):1317–9.
38. Vernois J, Redfern D, Ferraz L, et al. Minimally invasive surgery osteotomy of the hindfoot. Clin Podiatr Med Surg 2015;32(3):419–34.
39. Mitchell GP. Posterior displacement osteotomy of the calcaneus. J Bone Joint Surg Br 1977;59(2):233–5.

Endoscopic Resection of Tarsal Coalitions

Andrew King, MBChB, MRCS*, Stephen Parsons, MA, BS, FRCS, FRCS (Ed)

KEYWORDS

- Tarsal coalition • Talocalcaneal coalition • Calcaneonavicular coalition
- Arthroscopy • Endoscopy • Resection

KEY POINTS

- Endoscopic excision of both calcaneonavicular and talocalcaneal coalitions is technically feasible.
- Careful investigation preoperatively to understand each individual coalition is essential, particularly the extent of the joint involved in talocalcaneal coalitions.
- Consider the need for deformity correction alongside the resection of the coalition.
- Consider the need for posterior portals to resect talocalcaneal coalitions.
- More research is required to prove that endoscopic treatment of coalitions is more effective than open surgery.

INTRODUCTION

Tarsal coalition is a condition in which abnormal connections between tarsal bones are present.[1–3] These coalitions can be complete (bony) or incomplete fibro/cartilaginous. Coalitions result from failure of separation of mesenchymal tissue during embryologic development.[4]

INCIDENCE

The incidence of tarsal coalition has been reported between 1% and 6%,[1,2,5] although, because many coalitions are asymptomatic, the true incidence of this condition is likely to be higher. Cadaveric and imaging studies have suggested an incidence up to 13%.[6,7] There is a strong genetic predisposition with first-degree relatives often having a coalition that may well be asymptomatic.[8] Coalitions are bilateral in up to 50% of patients and are predominantly (>90%) talocalcaneal coalitions (TCC) or calcaneonavicular coalitions (CNC). Rarer types of tarsal coalitions are reported between the other tarsal bones.[9]

Trauma and Orthopaedics Department, Royal Cornwall Hospitals NHS Trust, Royal Cornwall Hospital, Treliske, Truro TR1 3LQ, UK
* Corresponding author.
E-mail address: andrewking3@nhs.net

Foot Ankle Clin N Am 25 (2020) 493–503
https://doi.org/10.1016/j.fcl.2020.05.009

foot.theclinics.com

CLINICAL PRESENTATION

Many coalitions will remain asymptomatic. In the authors' experience, patients from 3 differing groups can present with symptoms.

The first group is a presentation in late childhood or early adolescence with pain with or without deformity. Pain is typically located over the sinus tarsi for a CNC and beneath the medial malleolus for a TTC. Pain may also arise from soft tissue strain, muscle spasm, or extreme deformity. Patients may notice stiffness, although the gradual onset with progressive ossification may make its demonstration at examination a surprise. The classic deformity described in this condition is the planovalgus or flatfoot, but no deformity or even cavovarus can occur. The type and severity of deformity do not seem to consistently correlate with the type, position, size, or speed of ossification of the coalition. However, the age at which symptoms present appears to depend on the specific joints involved in the coalition and can range from 8 to 16 years.[10,11] According to Nalaboff and Schweitzer,[7] CNCs may present earlier, in children aged 8 to 12, compared with TCCs, which present in children between the ages of 12 and 16, because of the differing ages that ossification occurs at these sites.

The second group of patients is those in adolescence or early adult life who present with either a severe acute or recurrent chronic ankle sprains. Symptoms can be multifocal arising from the coalition or from the traumatic damage to ligaments or joints sustained from the injury. The damage may be greater than expected because of the stiffness arising from the previously asymptomatic coalition. Careful assessment and targeted investigations will be required to separate the sources of symptoms in this group, which may require differing treatments.

The final group presents as an adult of any age with symptoms arising from degenerative joint disease occurring as a secondary consequence of the altered joint function or deformity. Clinical examination and modern imaging techniques are required to determine which joints are affected because this will influence any subsequent joint-sacrificing surgery.[12,13]

DIAGNOSIS

Achieving a diagnosis begins with a clear history of the type, site, severity, and story of the symptoms and careful clinical examination of the stiffness of the joint and assessment of any deformity. Initial X rays should include weight-bearing ankle mortise, lateral foot and ankle, dorsoplantar, and non-weight-bearing oblique foot views. This latter view remains the gold standard for the CNC. The TCC may not be as clear with the X rays only showing an ill-defined middle facet, talar head spurring, or a "c" sign.

MRI is sensitive[14] for TCC and has the advantage of showing bone edema at the coalition but also any other areas of degenerative change and any unexpected pathologic condition. MRI can be useful in the group who present after a trauma.

When surgery is planned, computed tomography is beneficial for 3-dimensional (3D) imaging of deformity, but particularly for the site, shape, and size of a TCC. The classification by Rozansky and colleagues[15] is very helpful in operative planning.

TREATMENT

Treatment of tarsal coalition begins with conservative measures. These conservative measures can include rest, analgesics, and activity modification, with or without support from orthoses or bracing. Physiotherapy can be used to address foot flexibility or peroneal spasm. Steroid and local anesthetic injections can be used both diagnostically and therapeutically to the coalition or degenerate joints. Rest in a plaster cast or boot for 3 to 6 weeks may reduce symptoms.

In a retrospective analysis of nonoperative methods, a recent study has found 53% of 81 coalitions benefited from pain relief, and 70% of these coalitions avoided surgical intervention over the mean 19.8-month follow-up.[16] These findings were restricted to adolescents, and nonoperative treatment may be less successful in an adult because of the variety of underlying causes of the pain.[17]

Patients complaining of persistent, significant pain and diminished function despite thorough nonoperative measures can be considered for surgical intervention. Badgley[18] first described the open resection of a CNC in the 1920s. Fusion was initially more frequently used for TCCs because of the higher prevalence of degenerative changes in the subtalar joint at presentation.[19] Later studies proposed that resection of TCCs could be effective if the coalition was detected early.[20,21] There has been significant debate in the literature over whether and what to use as an interposition graft at the resection site.[3,12] Lemley and colleagues[22] suggested that there was no benefit in using an interposition graft. Aldahshan and colleagues[23] proposed that, for TCCs, if less than 50% of the joint surface is affected and in the absence of degenerative changes, resection should be attempted. Although most studies are case series, it appears outcomes for resection especially in younger patients with smaller coalitions can be favorable.[17,24]

All surgery, of any type, is planned directed damage, and open surgery involves unavoidable collateral damage to the tissues around the operated area. This unavoidable collateral damage increases the risks of pain, infection, scarring, and neuroma formation, and the healing of the open wound prolongs recovery. Endoscopic procedures aim to achieve the planned objective with less unnecessary collateral damage. They are only appropriate if the desired procedure can be achieved with equal or better effect and no greater risk of complications. These procedures thus have the potential benefits of reduced local trauma and faster recovery while reducing scarring over the foot and potentially interfering with any future surgical options.[24–28] Ankle joint arthroscopy was performed in the 1970s by pioneers such as Watanabe.[29] Since then, techniques and technology have improved to allow arthroscopy of the smaller joints of the foot. Van Dijk and colleagues[30] described the posterior portals for the ankle and subtalar joints. The sinus tarsi approach has allowed visualization of the anterior and middle calcaneal facets, talonavicular, and calcaneocuboid joints. The sinus tarsi approach was first applied to CNC in 2006 by Lui[25] and to TCC by Bonasia and colleagues[26] in 2011. Since this time, several case series have been published, but no randomized comparative trials have yet been performed.

CALCANEONAVICULAR COALITIONS

Since Lui[25] first described the technique for endoscopic CNC resection, there have been 6 case reports and case series reported in the literature. Bernardino and colleagues[27] published an experimental study in 2009 using cadaveric specimens and subsequently applied the technique to a single case of a 12-year-old patient. They sited their portals 3 to 4 mm anterior to the calcaneocuboid joint and medial to the extensor tendons in line with the calcaneocuboid joint but were forced to move this anteriorly because of the anatomic nature of the coalition. Successful resection was achieved and confirmed on 3D imaging. The American Orthopaedic Foot and Ankle Society (AOFAS) score for this patient was 98 at 10 weeks and 100 at 1 year. Iatrogenic resection of some bone beneath the anterior subtalar joint was noticed. In 2010, Bauer and colleagues[31] reported a single case of endoscopic resection of a CNC in an adult.

They recommended siting the viewing portal just dorsal to the angle of Gissane, and the working portal was sited based on the patient's anatomy using fluoroscopic guidance. They also noted degenerative changes at the talar head, which were debrided. The patient's AOFAS score improved from 23 to 82 at 2 years. In 2011, Knorr and colleagues[32] reported 3 cases with 12-month follow-up. Mean AOFAS scores increased from 58 preoperatively to 91 postoperatively. Nehme[33] reported a case study of endoscopic resection of bilateral CNCs in a 13-year-old patient. Similar portal placements were used as in previous studies, and the patient's AOFAS score was 82 two years postoperatively. The authors' own initial case series published in 2012[34] reported 4 cases of adolescents or young adults undergoing this procedure. Mean Manchester-Oxford Foot Questionnaire (MOXFQ) scores improved from 64.67 preoperatively to 25.33 postoperatively. The viewing portal was placed just dorsal to the angle of Gissane, and the working portal 5 mm dorsal and 1 to 1.5 cm distal over the coalition was confirmed on fluoroscopy. The largest case series to date was published by Bourlez and colleagues.[35] Eleven feet in 10 pediatric patients were studied using a similar surgical technique to other studies. Mean AOFAS scores improved 61.9 to 89.1 at a mean of 15 months. Complications noted during this study included persistent pain (2 patients), fibular tendinopathy (3 patients), postoperative hematoma (3 patients), and persistent subjective instability (3 patients). No neurovascular injuries have been reported in these studies. No recurrence has been noted, but there is significant variation in how this was assessed postoperatively; the length of follow-up is relatively short in all series. The outcomes of the above studies are shown in **Table 1**.

TALOCALCANEAL COALITIONS

Bonasia and colleagues[26] were the first to describe arthroscopic resection of TCCs in 2011. The investigators proposed that the posterior aspect of the coalition was more easily accessed through a posterior approach using the posteromedial and posterolateral portals on either side of the Achilles tendon. The importance of keeping instrumentation lateral to the flexor hallucis longus muscle (FHL) tendon was emphasized to reduce the risk of damage to the neuromuscular bundle. No patient data were presented as part of this study.

A combined early experience from Cornwall and Bristol was published in 2013.[36] This combined early experience reported the arthroscopic resection of middle facet

Table 1			
Summary of studies: endoscopic calcaneonavicular coalition resection			
Study	**No. of Cases**	**Follow-up (mo)**	**Outcomes**
Bernardino et al,[27] 2009	1	24	AOFAS 55 → 91
Bauer et al,[31] 2010	1	24	AOFAS 23 → 82
Knörr et al,[32] 2011	3	12	AOFAS 58 → 91
Singh & Parsons,[34] 2012	3	6	MOXFQ 64.67 → 25.33
Nehme et al,[33] 2016	1	24	AOFAS 82 postoperatively
Bourlez et al,[35] 2018	11	15	AOFAS 61.9 → 89.1

Data from Refs.[27,31–35]

coalitions with limited posterior extension onto the posterior facet. Clinical outcomes of 8 feet were recorded in 7 patients ranging from 13 to 20 years of age. The coalition was approached using 2 portals in the sinus tarsi. Having identified the distal extent of the coalition, arthroscopic resection then proceeded posteriorly under direct vision. Preoperative imaging delineating the shape and extent of the coalition was important. The Sports Athlete Foot and Ankle Score (SAFAS) was used in conjunction with a visual analogue scale (VAS) for pain. VAS improved from a preoperative level of 7.9 to 3.6 at a mean follow-up of 15 months. The SAFAS improved in all domains with the most improvement in sports performance. The authors observed 1 posterior tibial nerve injury in their study, and 1 patient went on to undergo bilateral subtalar fusions because of deterioration in symptoms and evidence of degenerative changes.

Hayashi and colleagues[37] reported the technique of posteromedial arthroscopy of the subtalar joint to resect both middle and posterior facet coalitions, although no patient data were presented in this publication. They describe using a viewing portal posterior to the medial malleolus and a working portal distal to the medial malleolus and a Cobb rasp to release the soft tissue creating a working space for resection. They highlight the dangers of tendon damage using this approach, but the potential advantages of being able to directly address the coalition, including posterior and middle facets. This technique has also been presented at the AOFAS annual meeting in 2016.[38] Three cases were reported with improvement in the AOFAS score from 65.3 to 92.3, but the timeframe for this is not recorded. No complications were recorded.

Knörr and colleagues[28] published a series of 16 feet in 2015 using the posterior approach. Coalitions were classified using the Rozansky method and were all middle facet coalitions without posterior extension. A textile band to retract the FHL tendon was used to increase visualization of the coalition, and a tunnel was then created through to the coalition, leaving a shell of medial bone to protect the soft tissues, which was then resected at the end of the procedure. Four patients in this series had an associated arthroereisis procedure for planovalgus deformity. Mean follow-up was 28 months, and AOFAS scores improved from 56.8 preoperatively to 90.9 postoperatively. One case of complex regional pain syndrome was reported with no other complications documented.

The largest series in the published literature is by Aldahshan and colleagues[23] in 2018. They reported 20 feet with a mean follow-up of 26 months. Again, using a nylon tape, the FHL tendon was retracted to give access to the middle facet. Mean AOFAS scores improved from 57.7 to 92.4 postoperatively. One patient was reported to have hyperesthesia 3 months postoperatively, which resolved, and no other complications were noted.

CORNWALL CURRENT TREATMENT PROTOCOLS
Calcaneonavicular Coalition

In the appropriately symptomatic patient who has not responded to conservative treatment, with a confirmed coalition on oblique X ray and no degenerative changes on scanning, endoscopic resection can be considered. Due consideration is given to the assessment of deformity because additional surgery may have to be considered for its correction. Patients whose symptoms from degenerative changes are sufficiently severe would normally be offered salvage surgery by arthroscopic subtalar or triple arthrodesis as appropriate.

The excision procedure is performed under general anesthesia with a supplementary local anesthetic ankle block and a thigh tourniquet. The patient is placed in a 45° "saggy" lateral position whereby the torso and the pelvis are supported halfway between supine and a full lateral position, with the uppermost limb placed on a firm foam pillow with the foot just hanging off its edge. No traction is required. A radiolucent operating table is used to allow for imaging. Important landmarks are identified and marked, outlining the sinus tarsi (**Fig. 1**).

The primary visualization portal is slightly dorsal to the angle of Gissane. The second working portal is placed 1 to 2 cm distal and 5 mm dorsal to the viewing portal overlying the calcanei-navicular coalition, confirming position with a needle, and fluoroscopy, if necessary (**Fig. 2**). Care is taken to protect the branches of the superficial peroneal and sural nerves when dissecting the portals by using the "nick-and-spread" technique.

A 3.5-mm 30° arthroscope is introduced at the viewing portal and a soft tissue shaver through the working portal to resect sufficient soft tissue to allow visibility (**Fig. 3**). The resection of coalition is performed with 3.5- and 4.5-mm bone-resecting burrs, from calcaneum to navicular and from lateral to medial. The resection is adequate when sufficient coalition has been excised all the way through to the medial soft tissues to produce a clear wide gap between the anterior process of the calcaneum and the navicular on direct vision and fluoroscopy (**Figs. 4** and **5**). The foot is assessed for any impingement between the anteromedial aspect of the calcaneus and the plantar lateral talar head on inversion and eversion movements. A bleeding point is commonly seen medially and benefits from electrocautery.

The patient's foot is wrapped in a wool and crepe bandage (no cast) before the tourniquet is released. The bandages are removed at 48 hours. Ankle and subtalar movements are strongly encouraged to start immediately postoperatively, especially while the regional block is still active. Elevation for 2 weeks is recommended to reduce bleeding, hematoma formation, and swelling. Partial weight-bearing is permitted immediately, increasing after 2 weeks guided by the level of pain.

Talocalcaneal Coalition

In the appropriate symptomatic patient who has not responded to conservative treatment, with predominantly a middle facet coalition on scanning and no degenerative

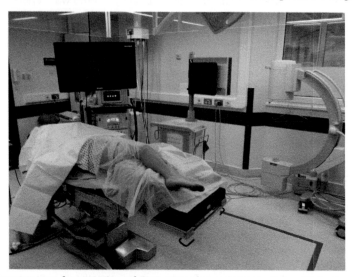

Fig. 1. Theater setup for resection of CNC. Note the endoscopy stack and the image intensifier positioning on the same side of the patient, who is positioned in the "saggy lateral" position. For a talonavicular coalition, the position would be "saggy prone."

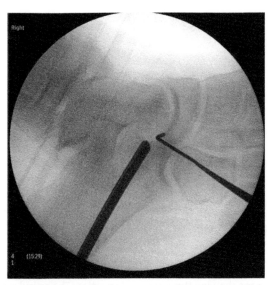

Fig. 2. Fluoroscopic image showing the instruments after creation of the portals for a CNC resection.

changes, arthroscopic resection can be considered. Again, deformity has to be carefully assessed because additional surgery may have to be considered for correction. Patients with very large coalitions or severe symptoms arising from degenerative changes would normally be offered arthroscopic subtalar or triple arthrodesis as appropriate.

The procedure is undertaken under general anesthesia with a supplementary local anesthetic ankle block and a thigh tourniquet. The patient is positioned on a

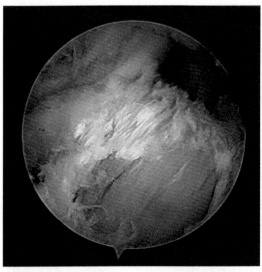

Fig. 3. Endoscopic image showing the coalition before resection: a soft tissue "pocket" has been created.

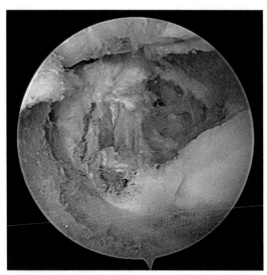

Fig. 4. Endoscopic image showing the completed resection. The articular cartilage of the talar head is visible in the top left and of the cuboid in the bottom right.

radiolucent operating table in the "recovery" or "saggy prone" position, whereby the torso is lateral and the pelvis is fixed halfway between prone and a full lateral position with the affected limb placed uppermost on a firm foam pillow. No traction is required. This position allows an approach to the coalition via the sinus tarsi with the foot in the lateral position, but also rotation of the limb to permit a posterior approach via the classical posterior portals.

The 2 standard portals are then made into the sinus tarsi. Sufficient fat and soft tissues are removed using a soft tissue shaver to produce visual clarity. The anterior

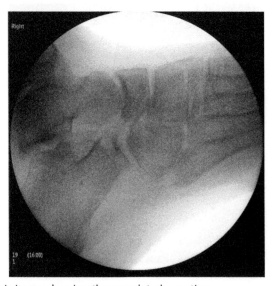

Fig. 5. Fluoroscopic image showing the completed resection.

edge of the posterior facet is followed to allow visualization of the middle facet. The coalition is fully delineated, and its distal extreme is exposed. The coalition is then excised using 3.5- and 4.5-mm arthroscopic barrel burrs. Because middle facet coalitions can be oblique rather than horizontal, resection is from dorsal to caudal, lateral to medial, and distal to proximal so as not to miss any extension into the posterior facet on the medial side. Great care is necessary on the posteromedial extent of the coalition because of the proximity of the posterior tibial nerve. Once the coalition has been fully excised, free subtalar movements at the posterior facet are confirmed clinically, arthroscopically, and radiologically before the portals are closed. If preoperative imaging indicates that the coalition extends significantly posteriorly or if the surgeon is unsure that the posterior extent of the coalition has been resected, then the posterior approach is used to complete the procedure.

Postoperatively, patients are managed in a similar manner to those undergoing CNC resection.

SUMMARY

Endoscopic excision of tarsal coalitions is technically feasible, and experience with these techniques is accumulating. However, careful investigation and consideration of the individual case are necessary before proceeding with this technique. First, exclusion of degenerative changes in the affected or surrounding joints is necessary. Second, the requirement for deformity correction must be assessed and the effect of additional procedures on the surgery must be considered. Third, particularly in patients presenting with trauma, alternative causes of pain must be excluded before treating the coalition. Finally, particularly when treating TCCs, the extent of the coalition should be fully defined and the surgical approach to it considered.

Excision of a CNC is more straightforward than a TCC, and hence, more series exist in the literature for the former technique. Evidence for the efficacy of endoscopic resection of tarsal coalitions is limited. There is an impression that pain is reduced and recovery is faster, but this is far from proven. Comparative trials to investigate this further would be useful. There is also a paucity of long-term follow-up for patients having undergone these procedures, and recurrence rates are not known nor is the effect of the lack of interposition material in these techniques. Further research is certainly required in this area.

DISCLOSURE

The authors have nothing to disclose.

REFERENCES

1. Zaw H, Calder JDF. Tarsal coalitions. Foot Ankle Clin 2010;15:349–64.

2. Wray JB, Nash Herndon C. Hereditary transmission of congenital coalition of the calcaneus to the navicular. J Bone Joint Surg 1963;45(2):365–72.

3. Klammer G, Espinosa N, Iselin LD. Coalitions of the tarsal bones. Foot Ankle Clin 2018;23:435–49.

4. Leonard MA. The inheritance of tarsal coalition and its relationship to spastic flat foot. J Bone Joint Surg Br 1974;56B:520–6.

5. Lysack JT, Fenton PV. Variations in calcaneonavicular morphology demonstrated with radiography. Radiology 2004;230:493–7.

6. Rühli FJ, Solomon LB, Henneberg M. High prevalence of tarsal coalitions and tarsal joint variants in a recent cadaver sample and its possible significance. Clin Anat 2003;16:411–5.

7. Nalaboff KM, Schweitzer ME. MRI of tarsal coalition: frequency, distribution, and innovative signs. Bull NYU Hosp Jt Dis 2008;66:14–21.

8. Docquier P-L, Maldaque P, Bouchard M. Tarsal coalition in paediatric patients. Orthop Traumatol Surg Res 2019;105:S123–31.

9. Lawrence DA, Rolen MF, Haims AH, et al. Tarsal coalitions: radiographic, CT, and MR imaging findings. HSS J 2014;10:153–66.

10. Mosca VS. Subtalar coalition in pediatrics. Foot Ankle Clin 2015;20:265–81.

11. Katayama T, Tanaka Y, Kadono K, et al. Talocalcaneal coalition: a case showing the ossification process. Foot Ankle Int 2005;26:490–3.

12. Zhou B, Tang K, Hardy M. Talocalcaneal coalition combined with flatfoot in children: diagnosis and treatment: a review. J Orthop Surg Res 2014;9:129.

13. Varner KE, Michelson JD. Tarsal coalition in adults. Foot Ankle Int 2000;21: 669–72.

14. Guignand D, Journeau P, Mainard-Simard L, et al. Child calcaneonavicular coalitions: MRI diagnostic value in a 19-case series. Orthop Traumatol Surg Res 2011;97:67–72.

15. Rozansky A, Varley E, Moor M, et al. A radiologic classification of talocalcaneal coalitions based on 3D reconstruction. J Child Orthop 2010;4:129–35.

16. Shirley E, Gheorghe R, Neal KM. Results of nonoperative treatment for symptomatic tarsal coalitions. Cureus 2018;10:e2944.

17. Flynn JF, Wukich DK, Conti SF, et al. Subtalar coalitions in the adult. Foot Ankle Clin 2015;20:283–91.

18. Badgley CE. Coalition of the calcaneus and the navicular. Arch Surg 1927; 15(1):75.

19. Cowell HR. Talocalcaneal coalition and new causes of peroneal spastic flatfoot. Clin Orthop Relat Res 1972;85:16–22.

20. Wilde PH, Torode IP, Dickens DR, et al. Resection for symptomatic talocalcaneal coalition. J Bone Joint Surg Br 1994;76:797–801.

21. Scranton PE Jr. Treatment of symptomatic talocalcaneal coalition. J Bone Joint Surg Am 1987;69:533–9.

22. Lemley F, Berlet G, Hill K, et al. Current concepts review: tarsal coalition. Foot Ankle Int 2006;27:1163–9.

23. Aldahshan W, Hamed A, Elsherief F, et al. Endoscopic resection of different types of talocalcaneal coalition. Foot Ankle Int 2018;39:1082–8.

24. Luhmann SJ, Schoenecker PL. Symptomatic talocalcaneal coalition resection: indications and results. J Pediatr Orthop 1998;18:748–54.

25. Lui TH. Arthroscopic resection of the calcaneonavicular coalition or the "too long" anterior process of the calcaneus. Arthroscopy 2006;22:903.e1-4.

26. Bonasia DE, Phisitkul P, Saltzman CL, et al. Arthroscopic resection of talocalcaneal coalitions. Arthroscopy 2011;27:430–5.

27. Bernardino CM, Golanó P, Garcia MA, et al. Experimental model in cadavera of arthroscopic resection of calcaneonavicular coalition and its first in-vivo application: preliminary communication. J Pediatr Orthop B 2009;18:347.

28. Knörr J, Soldado F, Menendez ME, et al. Arthroscopic talocalcaneal coalition resection in children. Arthroscopy 2015;31:2417–23.

29. Watanabe M. Selfoc-arthroscope (Watanabe No. 24 arthroscope) (monograph). Tokyo: Teishin Hospital; 1972.

30. van Dijk CN, Scholten PE, Krips R. A 2-portal endoscopic approach for diagnosis and treatment of posterior ankle pathology. Arthroscopy 2000;16:871–6.

31. Bauer T, Golano P, Hardy P. Endoscopic resection of a calcaneonavicular coalition. Knee Surg Sports Traumatol Arthrosc 2010;18:669–72.

32. Knörr J, Accadbled F, Abid A, et al. Arthroscopic treatment of calcaneonavicular coalition in children. Orthop Traumatol Surg Res 2011;97:565–8.

33. Nehme AH, Bou Monsef J, Bou Ghannam AG, et al. Arthroscopic resection of a bilateral calcaneonavicular coalition in a child. J Foot Ankle Surg 2016;55(5): 1079–82.

34. Singh AK, Parsons SW. Arthroscopic resection of calcaneonavicular coalition/malunion via a modified sinus tarsi approach: an early case series. Foot Ankle Surg 2012;18:266–9.

35. Bourlez J, Joly-Monrigal P, Alkar F, et al. Does arthroscopic resection of a too-long anterior process improve static disorders of the foot in children and adolescents? Int Orthop 2018;42:1307–12.

36. Jagodzinski NA, Hughes A, Davis NP, et al. Arthroscopic resection of talocalcaneal coalitions: a bicentre case series of a new technique. Foot Ankle Surg 2013; 19(2):125–30.

37. Hayashi K, Kumai T, Tanaka Y. Endoscopic resection of a talocalcaneal coalition using a posteromedial approach. Arthrosc Tech 2014;e39–43.

38. Nakazora S, Nishimura A, Ito N, et al. Endoscopic resection for talocalcaneal coalition using posteromedial approach. Foot & Ankle Orthopaedics 2016. https://doi.org/10.1177/2473011416s00064. 2473011416S0006.

Moving?

Make sure your subscription moves with you!

To notify us of your new address, find your **Clinics Account Number** (located on your mailing label above your name), and contact customer service at:

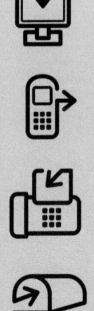

Email: journalscustomerservice-usa@elsevier.com

800-654-2452 (subscribers in the U.S. & Canada)
314-447-8871 (subscribers outside of the U.S. & Canada)

Fax number: 314-447-8029

Elsevier Health Sciences Division
Subscription Customer Service
3251 Riverport Lane
Maryland Heights, MO 63043

*To ensure uninterrupted delivery of your subscription, please notify us at least 4 weeks in advance of move.

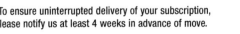

Printed and bound by CPI Group (UK) Ltd, Croydon, CR0 4YY

03/10/2024

01040407-0013